Love, Sex and Psychoth
in a Post-Romantic Era

How do cultural changes such as the increasing lustful possibilities of our liquid modernity affect 'romantic' values as psychotherapists and counsellors – and, in turn, affect how they work through their clients' relationships? Do they embody values from a previous era that are inappropriate for the era we are in now, which some term 'post-romantic'? For example, do they really privilege monogamous relationships? There again, do those psychotherapists who advocate polygamy really want others to legitimize their own desires to have affairs? How wary should one be of accepting such prevailing theories as Freud's nuclear family romance and his 'ordinary unhappiness'? Is anyone value-free regarding romanticism/post-romanticism and should they be? Is 'to have and to hold from this day forward, for better for worse, for richer or poorer, in sickness and in health, to love and to cherish, till death us do part' still an ideal worth working towards or more an ideological imprisonment? This book seeks to explore recent research on how notions of romanticism and post-romanticism affect therapeutic practices.

Love, Sex and Psychotherapy in a Post-Romantic Era is a significant new contribution to psychotherapy, and will be a great resource for prospective and current clients, trainee and professional therapists, academics, researchers and advanced students of psychology, psychotherapy, philosophy and human behaviour.

This book was originally published as a special issue of the *European Journal of Psychotherapy & Counselling*.

Del Loewenthal is Emeritus Professor of Psychotherapy and Counselling at the University of Roehampton, London, UK, and Chair of SAFPAC (www.safpac.co.uk). He is an existential-analytic psychotherapist, photographer and chartered psychologist, with a particular interest in phenomenology (www.delloewenthal.com). His books include *Existential Psychotherapy and Counselling after Postmodernism* (2017).

Love, Sex and Psychotherapy in a Post-Romantic Era

Edited by
Del Loewenthal

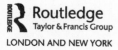

Routledge
Taylor & Francis Group

LONDON AND NEW YORK

First published 2021
by Routledge
2 Park Square, Milton Park, Abingdon, Oxon OX14 4RN

and by Routledge
52 Vanderbilt Avenue, New York, NY 10017

First issued in paperback 2022

Routledge is an imprint of the Taylor & Francis Group, an informa business

British Library Cataloguing in Publication Data
A catalogue record for this book is available from the British Library

Typeset in Minion
by Newgen Publishing UK

Publisher's Note
The publisher accepts responsibility for any inconsistencies that may have arisen during the conversion of this book from journal articles to book chapters, namely the inclusion of journal terminology.

Disclaimer
Every effort has been made to contact copyright holders for their permission to reprint material in this book. The publishers would be grateful to hear from any copyright holder who is not here acknowledged and will undertake to rectify any errors or omissions in future editions of this book.

ISBN 13: 978-0-367-56120-8 (pbk)
ISBN 13: 978-0-367-56119-2 (hbk)

Contents

Citation Information

The chapters in this book were originally published in the *European Journal of Psychotherapy & Counselling*, volume 21, issue 3-4 (2019). When citing this material, please use the original page numbering for each article, as follows:

Chapter 1

Should love be unconditional?
Helen Gilbert
European Journal of Psychotherapy & Counselling, volume 21, issue 3-4 (2019), pp. 194–204

Chapter 2

Romance and murder
Sally Parsloe
European Journal of Psychotherapy & Counselling, volume 21, issue 3-4 (2019), pp. 205–216

Chapter 3

Polyamory - a romantic solution to wanderlust?
Marian O'Connor
European Journal of Psychotherapy & Counselling, volume 21, issue 3-4 (2019), pp. 217–230

Chapter 4

A phenomenology of love, thanks to Lacan, Miller, and Jellybean
Tony McSherry
European Journal of Psychotherapy & Counselling, volume 21, issue 3-4 (2019), pp. 231–243

Chapter 5

Conversations outside the walls of the city: Techniques, erotic love and the wings of desire in Phaedrus *and psychotherapy*
Onel Brooks
European Journal of Psychotherapy & Counselling, volume 21, issue 3-4 (2019), pp. 244–262

For any permission-related enquiries please visit:
www.tandfonline.com/page/help/permissions

Notes on Contributors

Onel Brooks, Southern Association for Psychotherapy and Counselling and Research Group for Therapeutic Education, University of Roehampton, London, UK.

Christopher Clulow, Tavistock Institute of Medical Psychology, London, UK.

Helen Gilbert, Southern Association for Psychotherapy and Counselling and Research Group for Therapeutic Education, University of Roehampton, London, UK.

Del Loewenthal, Southern Association for Psychotherapy and Counselling and Research Group for Therapeutic Education, University of Roehampton, London, UK.

Tony McSherry, Southern Association for Psychotherapy and Counselling and Research Group for Therapeutic Education, University of Roehampton, London, UK.

Marian O'Connor, Psychoanalytic Couple Psychotherapist, Psychosexual Therapist, Head of Psychosexual Training at Tavistock Relationships, London, UK.

Sally Parsloe, Southern Association for Psychotherapy and Counselling and Research Group for Therapeutic Education, University of Roehampton, London, UK.

Poul Rohleder, Department of Psychosocial and Psychoanalytic Studies, University of Essex, Colchester, UK.

Paola Valerio, Research Group for Therapeutic Education, University of Roehampton, London, UK.

Introduction: Love, sex and psychotherapy in a post-romantic era – Whatever happened to the magic of the relational?

Del Loewenthal

'Last Saturday night I thought I would try "aggressive African", at least that's what he calls it on the website. It wasn't actually that aggressive and he was alright really; but he was only a student.' This client, who men seem to find attractive and who is considered to be good at sex texting and doing it 'as on the porn sites' has come to therapy as she longs to be able to marry sex and intimacy.

In various ways, we do seem to be in an era of more sexual freedoms. Is this part of Bauman's *Liquid Modernity* (2000), where individuals can shift from one sexual orientation to another excluding themselves from traditional networks of support such as family, while also freeing themselves from the restrictions or requirements those networks impose? Furthermore, what of those such as Lucy Irigaray (1985) who write that sexual difference is to do with language and culture rather than biology? Irigaray (1993) further argues that we are in an age of sexual difference which is founded, and here she agrees with Lacan, in language.[1] Yet there would also appear to be a neo-traditional turn among young people, epitomised by the popularity of Jordan Peterson (2019), where 'fluidity' is being rejected, and people are looking for commitment.

Certainly, the pace of relational change would appear to be rapidly increasing for many with, for example, the recent announcement of the closure in the UK of the ground-breaking Women's Therapy Centre (womenstherapycentre.com) yet growing concerns with men's mental health giving rise to such developments as my own involvement in re-establishing the Men's Therapy Centre (menstherapycentre.com). However, has there for example ever been a relatively better time, at least in living memory, to be LGBTQ+? Yet, Samuel Adamson in his play *Wife* (2019) implies, as Billington (2019) puts it, that 'we are still wrestling with the problem Ibsen [in *A Doll's House*]… confronted in a pioneering way: how to balance personal freedoms with equality in relationships'. There is also, as Pleck (2000) argues, people being left disappointed because they buy into an idea of fulfilment through one partner, who typically does not live up to these overly embellished expectations. It would, therefore, appear there is increasing acceptance of those who are LGBTQ+ as part of our society with, for example, what appears to be a growing number of people identifying as bisexual as well as children and those around them considering themselves not to be gender-stereotypical. Surely this is more than helpful to many? There again, could it be disastrous for those who are no longer allowed to work through what can be seen as vital developmental stages? Yet besides such conflicting ideas regarding the relative dangers of over-encouraging those growing up, in the name of necessary education, could such changes also be at the expense of love and intimacy in our overall culture? Indeed, whatever happened to, what at least some of us thought was, *the magic of the relational* (Loewenthal 2014: 3–11)?

Would it be wrong to associate the loosening of sexual mores with similar historical times such as Germany's Weimar Republic (with Christopher Isherwood's *Goodbye to Berlin* [1989], Fritz Lang's *Metropolis* [1927], Otto Dix's paintings, etc.)? We do seem currently to be increasingly wearing the fashion colours of that time and while it would be wrong to make a direct comparison with Hitler, we seem, at least in the USA and UK, to be electing populist politicians who are able to openly be unfaithful and blatantly untruthful. While this might be seen as attempts to return to an imperial past in order not to acknowledge the decline of the West, it would seem to both be brought about by, and contribute to, our increasing inability to come to our senses. We are seeing a growth in anti-semitism, and through populism the poor are being duped into voting for tax cuts for the oligarchs, etc. What chance then for the abilities of psychotherapists (who are increasingly part of the general culture rather than being more subversively outside of it) to come to their own senses let alone help the client/patient with theirs? Otherwise, perhaps increasingly we will be 'making use of' our new post-romantic sexual freedoms by, to give a further example, taking part in the extraordinary growth in the 'sugar daddy' industry (seeking.arrangement. com) which claims to have over 500,000 UK students signed up, luring them with such legitimising normalising claims as 'being great for networking', as reported in BBC TV's (2019) *Secrets of Sugar Baby Dating*. This might be seen as part of a reappraisal of existing relationships as in Zelizer (2007), *The Purchase of Intimacy*. Here she argues that it is taboo to view money and intimacy as entangled but they in fact often are, whether it be in parental or romantic love or in more crude (but she would say, equivalent) forms such as the sugar daddy industry.

Post-romanticism is increasingly being seen as an important way of exploring what is changing in our lives with regard to love, sex and intimacy. In contrast, in romanticism, which developed from the 18th century:

> We are introduced to nameless longing, to mystery and the unsayable. Romanticism, with the love of the fragment, the sketch, the unfinished, the merely suggestive... It involves us as co-creators... with responsibilities... for ourselves and each other...
>
> (Snell 2017: 174)

Post-romanticism, as in the title of this book, considers whether relationships after the initial 'romanticism' should be sustained, and if yes, then how? The question here is to what extent, if any, are other sexual relations more permissible in what is being termed a post-romantic era? Alain de Botton (2016) in *How Romanticism Ruined Love* argues that romanticism is a disaster for relationships and that we need to realise that love and sex do not always belong together. Rather, we need to have a post-romantic future for love.

What then are our views on, for example, in the UK the current growing trend of popular BBC television series as *Strictly Come Dancing* with its '*Strictly* curse' of evolving sexual relations or *Wanderlust*'s explorations of polygamy? Or, even more 'in your face', ITV2's most popular ever programme, *Love Island*. The format here (now franchised to many countries) is that on the first day, the Islanders couple up for the first time based on first impressions, but over the duration of the series they are forced to 're-couple' where they can choose to remain in their current couple or swap and change (some of these contestants, and the presenter, have subsequently committed suicide). The viewer can see these couplings' processes to the extent of watching sexual intercourse taking place in a bedroom full of double beds. To go back in history again, is this similar (as with our increasing fixations with TV programmes such as *Game of Thrones*) to when the Roman Emperors had to think up even more ghastly scenes for the populace to be drawn to the Colosseum in order to take their minds off their direly oppressive situation?

So is post-romanticism a growing worldwide trend or are the above examples more specific to parts of the UK where, as the OECD (2019) report shows, Britain is second bottom in rankings of young people claiming their life has purpose and perhaps an alienation from their bodies and hearts if they cannot have meaningful sexual relationships. This would not seem to be the case from an ethnography (Sirisena 2018) of university students in Sri Lanka where love and companionship appear highly sought after as a source of continuity. Nor, to give one more example, where it is reported (Ahearn 2001) that romanticism has affected Hinduism in Nepal, as young people find the idea of a romantic love compelling.

Yet, how do such cultural changes, affect the 'romantic', or otherwise, values of psychotherapists and counsellors; and, in turn, affect how they work with their clients/patients regarding their relationships? Do they embody values from a previous era that are inappropriate for the current era, which some term 'post-romantic'? For example, do they really privilege monogamous relationships? There again, do those psychotherapists who advocate polygamy really want others to legitimise their own desire to have affairs? How wary should we be of accepting such prevailing theories as Freud's nuclear family romance and his 'ordinary unhappiness' (2004)? Are we value-free regarding romanticism/post-romanticism and should we be? Is 'to have and to hold from this day forward, for better for worse, for richer or poorer, in sickness and in health, to love and to cherish, till death us do part' (Church of England,

2019) still an ideal worth working towards or more an ideological imprisonment? This book seeks to explore recent research on how our notions of romanticism and post-romanticism affect our therapeutic practices and I will now introduce the forthcoming chapters.

Chapter 1 'Should love be unconditional?' is by Helen Gilbert. Here, Helen argues that to see love between parents and children as conditional and therefore breakable, optional and vulnerable is a taboo. One of the peer reviewers of this chapter commented: 'Overall there is a freshness to the paper rather than over-theorising or intellectualising the content and thereby deadening it'.

Chapter 2 'Romance and murder' is by Sally Parsloe. Sally presents the interesting view that romance is essentially an adult form of fairy tale which serves the same purpose of processing of conflicts and trauma but runs the risk of turning murderous when the image created 'threatens to have a life of its own'. Difficulties we face in our adult life which link back to our earlier childhood experiences are highlighted. A case is presented which illustrates this view.

Marian O'Connor provides our third chapter entitled 'Polyamory – a romantic solution to wanderlust?' This chapter can be seen to engage with the topic of polyamory in a careful and unprejudiced way, illustrating both its psychological and social advantages and disadvantages. Importantly, it provides thoughtful guidelines and case material for practitioners who work with polyamorous individuals, couples or triads. In so doing, the author offers us her views on the technical challenges for therapists who work with polyamorous individuals and relationships.

Next in Chapter 4, Anthony McSherry in 'A phenomenology of love, thanks to Lacan, Miller, and Jellybean' provides an account of love and the brokenhearted. Here the author invites us to consider whether rather than just phenomenologically staying with experience, or alternatively taking refuge in theory, we can explore such Lacanian notions as love being like 'a maze of misunderstandings with no exit' in helping us understand, for example, Jellybean's importance.

Chapter 5, 'Conversations outside the walls of the city: Techniques, erotic love and the wings of desire in *Phaedrus* and psychotherapy', is by Onel Brooks. Here, Onel explores the issue of the balance – or conflict – between order and control on one side, and passion and commitment on the other. This theme is developed in the context of the client, the therapist, and Plato's *Phaedrus*. The author puts the case, through Socrates, of love not being something that we have under our control. Rather, it is something that might lead us, as Plato seemed to value it, to speaking about what is important to us: to companionship and conversation. As a reviewer pointed out, Onel's chapter touches on a subject that has significance beyond therapy as politicians seem again increasingly able through their speeches to arouse strong emotions which are at odds with the reasoned case for and against a course of action.

Chapter 6, 'Is Oedipus still blind: A countertransference take on love and hate in the consulting room', is by Paola Valerio. Paola addresses topics that can be seen as essential in widening our thinking about erotic transference and so-called countertransference and to address gender bias. The chapter is written in a manner that can evoke vivid imagery. The focus on counter-transference and the therapist's erotic and hateful feelings towards the patient is an interesting and fruitful one.

Chapter 7 is Poul Rohleder's published response on the above six chapters, which he entitles '(No) time for love: Reflecting on relationships in psycho-therapy'. Poul's chapter uniquely explores temporality in relation to these preceding chapters. He argues that psychoanalysis has never been a romantic endeavour. Rather, it recognises 'the role of being able to tolerate love and hatred in the experience of intimate relationships, whatever its forms'.

The second published respondent and final chapter is by Christopher Clulow. In his 'Love, sex and psychotherapy in a post-romantic age: A commentary', Christopher puts forward the idea of post-romanticism as a historical con-struction where all choices of a stable couple are post-romantic. He offers a sense that all individuals, regardless of their particular way of relating, to be able to arrive at a stable and satisfying relationship, have in common the cap-acity to emerge from 'the many minor deaths associated with enduring love'.

I would like to end this introduction with a further quote from this, what I regard as particularly illuminating, last review chapter:

> …we short-change ourselves and our patients if we lose sight of either heart or mind, and the significance of the objects to which they become attached. The act of loving is never conflict-free.

Perhaps with all the increasing lustful possibilities of our liquid modernity, the above quote is still worth considering. All the more so regarding balancing 'personal freedoms with equality in relationships' not only between couples but in our society as a whole – though some may see this as essential and others as an unnecessary traditional restriction.

I hope this book may help you to reconsider your views, whatever they are!

Notes

1 However, unlike Lacan, importantly Irigaray argues that the symbolic order is not ahistorical and unchanging; and she further disagrees that Lacan's phallic is ahistor-ical and not to do with male anatomy – hence more potential liquidity.

References

Abel, A., Fröhlich, G., George, H., Harbou, T. von, Helm, B., Klein-Rogge, R., Lang, F., Loos, T., & Pommer, E. (1927). *Metropolis*. New York, NY: Kino International
Adamson, S. (2019). *Wife*. London: Faber and Faber.

Ahearn, L. (2001). *Invitations to love literacy, love letters, and social change in Nepal*. Ann Arbor: University of Michigan Press.

Bauman, Z. (2000). *Liquid modernity*. Cambridge: Polity Press.

BBC TV. (2019, June 12). 'Secrets of sugar baby dating', retrieved from www.bbc.co.uk/iplayer/episode/p07bmxj3/secrets-of-sugar-baby-dating

Billington, M. (2019, June 5). 'Wife Review – Rousing look at 60 years of sexual identity', *The Guardian*.

Church of England. (2019). 'Marriage', retrieved from www.churchofengland.org/prayer-and-worship/worship-texts-and-resources/common-worship/marriage#mm093

de Botton, A. (2016). 'How romanticism ruined love', retrieved from https://www.abc.net.au/religion/how-romanticism-ruined-love/10096750

Freud, S., & Breuer, J. (2004). *Studies in hysteria*. London: Penguin Classics.

Irigary, L. (1985). *Speculum of the other woman*. Ithaca, NY: Cornell University Press.

Irigary, L. (1993). *Ethics of sexual difference*. Ithaca, NY: Cornell University Press.

Isherwood, C. (1989). *Goodbye to Berlin*. London: Vintage Classics.

Loewenthal, D. (2014). 'The magic of the relational' in Loewenthal, D., & Samuels, A. *Relational psychotherapy, psychoanalysis and counselling: Appraisals and reappraisals*. Abingdon: Routledge.

OECD (2019). *Education at a glance 2019: OECD indicators*. Paris: OECD Publishing.

Peterson, J. (2019). *12 Rules for life: An antidote for chaos*. London: Penguin.

Pleck, E. (2000). *Celebrating the family: Ethnicity, consumer culture and family rituals*. Cambridge, MA: Harvard University Press.

Sirisena, M. (2018). *Making and meaning of relationships in Sri Lanka*. London: Palgrave Macmillan.

Snell, R. (2017). *Portraits of the insane: Theodore Gericault and the subject of psychotherapy*. Abingdon: Routledge.

Zelizer, V. (2007). *The purchase of intimacy*. Princeton, NJ: Princeton University Press.

Should love be unconditional?

Helen Gilbert

ABSTRACT

This paper questions the idea that within families love should always be unconditional and raises the issue of family estrangement in the context of psychotherapy. It will look at whether there has been a generational shift towards individualism and consider how this affects the notion of love. Does the author respond to her clients from a belief that love should be unconditional or from a vicarious wish to be free from her own difficult family members? Is the therapeutic space available for the taboo of unconditional family love to be fully explored? The author will explore her experience as a psychological therapist working with people estranged from family in order to examine her own biases.Family relationships, as well as romantic relationships, are impacted by the culture we live in, and therapeutic relationships are affected by the therapist's unconscious and conscious biases. In response to the question posed the author concludes that love between adults is always conditional even if this is a truth we cannot fully accept. Although conditions on love may be seen as healthy in a romantic relationship, the bonds between family members are generally held up as sacrosanct and unbreakable. This makes the choice to walk away from family difficult for wider society, therapists and estranged individuals to bear.

This paper questions the idea that within families love should always be unconditional and raises the issue of family estrangement in the context of psychotherapy. It will look at whether there has been a generational shift towards individualism and consider how this affects the notion of love.

Does the author respond to her clients from a belief that love should be unconditional or from a vicarious wish to be free from her own difficult family members? Is the therapeutic space available for the taboo of unconditional family love to be fully explored? The author will explore her experience as a psychological therapist working with people estranged from family in order to examine her own biases.

Family relationships, as well as romantic relationships, are impacted by the culture we live in, and therapeutic relationships are affected by the therapist's unconscious and conscious biases. In response to the question posed the author concludes that love between adults is always conditional even if this is a truth we cannot fully accept. Although conditions on love may be seen as healthy in a romantic relationship, the bonds between family members are generally held up as sacrosanct and unbreakable. This makes the choice to walk away from family difficult for wider society, therapists and estranged individuals to bear.

"Loving is to give what one does not have to someone who doesn't want it"
(Lacan, 1965).

This paper questions the idea that within families love should always be unconditional and raises the issue of family estrangement in the context of psychotherapy and therapeutic support groups. The author, who is a psychotherapeutic counsellor examines what therapeutic space is available for the taboo that family love is conditional, optional and fragile to be fully explored. The author will also look at her experience as a psychological therapist working with people estranged from family in order to examine some of her own biases.

This paper starts from the assumption that love between family members is considered to be unconditional in a Western societal paradigm and, moreover, that the converse view, that love between a parent and child may be conditional and thus potentially breakable, is effectively taboo in our society. This assumption is based on the author's experience of working in the field of family estrangement and hearing first-hand about the stigma faced by people who choose or are subject to estrangement.

It is not simple to find one original meaning for the term unconditional love. This idea appears in the Bible to describe God's unconditional love for his people and the way in which they are told to love one another. In ancient Greek scholarship the word Agape is used to describe a sacrificial kind of love that is usually at cost to the bearer.

To problematize this idea, it could be argued that in the Judeo-Christian tradition God's love is not really unconditional at all. His love is based on the adherence of believers to a certain set of beliefs and behaviours. In order for believers to be saved and thus receive God's apparently unconditional love they must accept his view that they are sinful and believe and accept his forgiveness and truth about them. Perhaps it could be more honestly stated that unconditional love is a collective wish that we humans hold, which at the same time serves to repress the fear that we may not ever be fully loved.

According to research carried out by Stand Alone, a charity supporting people experiencing estrangement, 1 in 5 families in the UK will be affected by estrangement and over 5 million people have decided to cut contact with at least one family member. It could be argued that the prevalence of individualism since 1960's, along with increased divorce rates and greater agency for women have created a culture framed by the 'disposability of relationships' (Lebey, 2001), however, Agllias, a leading researcher in the field, argues that 'there is little evidence to suggest that estrangement is a new phenomenon' (Agllias, 2017).

Exploration of space available in support groups to explore feelings relating to estrangement

In her role running support groups for a national charity supporting people experiencing family estrangement, the author works with two distinct client groups, parents estranged from their children (of whatever age) and adult children estranged from their parents or siblings.

One of the support groups run with estranged parents elicited a feeling of helplessness in the author, who was the facilitator of the group. The group members were desperate to know how to get their adult children to come back, and seemingly longed for her to provide them with what seemed like, a magical solution that would bring about reconciliation. Creating space in a support group for feelings such as hopelessness and helplessness, desperation and deep grief to be shared could be seen as the main work of the group but this often proves very testing. In this group there seemed to be a strong resistance to sharing painful feelings. In each session one of the group members would ask if everyone could come up with a strategy to deal with estrangement and kept interrupting others when they got upset or spoke for too long. The rest of the group joined in with this way of behaving and would often say at the end of the session that they couldn't see the point in coming to the group as no-one (directed at the facilitator) was solving the estrangement. The facilitator tried to help the group members to look at their own part in what had happened in their families but the group narrative became focused on not knowing why their adult children had cut them off and blaming society for becoming too permissive and individualistic.

It felt as if the group was pushing the facilitator to reinforce their wishful belief in unconditional family love, meaning love as duty and love for the family over and above any personal need or desire. Several group members were angry that a way for their adult children to come back to them was not proffered. It could be considered that this group of parents were narcissistic in their attitudes towards their children. Anger was common to every session: anger that a solution to solve the situation was not forthcoming, anger that some in the group had accepted estrangement as a way of life, anger that the fact of familial roles is not enough to guarantee relationship. Sometimes anger dominated the group process but towards the end, one of the group members came to a realisation that condemning her daughter for not fulfilling her filial duty would not restore their relationship and may

instead push her further away. This seemingly calm and unemotional out-
burst opened up feelings of grief, guilt and shame in other group members.
This also brought out more compassion from group members towards one
another.

This observation brings to mind the notion that it seems to be more
painful to accept that wholeness and completeness do not exist and to
continue to seek the fantasy of unconditional love rather than to accept
the trauma of broken relationships along with the arguably healthier position of separateness. But this may be to conflate unconditional love and
a pre-Oedipal merged relationship. This leads to a question of whether
there is a different order of love that exists from parent to child than child
to parent. Perhaps unconditional love may only exist from a parent to
a child. Parental love is also different to any other as the relationship is
always working towards a separation or at least a partial separation. The
parent's role is to enable the child to grow up and become a separate
individual able to manage without their parents. This may inevitably
mean that they make different choices to their parents in terms of religion,
relationships, sex, education and career. All of these differences may provoke estrangement due to the difference or arguably the separation itself
becoming unacceptable. It may also be that separation itself is problematic
for some parents who struggle to accept that they are not still merged.

The author notes that her responses and biases have changed towards
estranged parents since identifying as a parent herself. When first working
with groups of parents estranged from their children, she was aware of her
own anger towards the group members, and identification with the
estranged children. She took the position of being the child of her own
anxious, self-absorbed parents in opposition to people who were demanding of unconditional love despite their judgemental, uncaring, very conditional attitude towards their children. Since becoming a parent and
returning to the work, the author recognises a personal shift towards
identification with the parents and greater compassion towards their pain
at being separated from their children.

It might be argued that this shift has allowed more psychic space to be
created in which painful feelings can be expressed about the loss of a child.
This is highlighted in feelings of greater compassion for the grieving
parents. Conversely, however, it sometimes seems to be the case that the
potential loss of a child feels too great and must be defended against; this is
shown when the facilitator joins in (internally at least) with casting blame
on the estranged parents rather than accepting that love between adults
may indeed have limits or conditions for both parties. This again leads to
the idea that it is less traumatic to retain a fantasy of perfect union between
parent and child or an ideal of unconditional love, even if it results in anger

and hurt towards self and other, rather than to accept that real love between adults may be more separate and conditional.

At the same time the author felt that she had to take up the position of the parent in a group of young children who were not able to recognise the experience or suffering of others. One could suppose that this observation may shed some light on the way that these group members parented their own children, which may be a potential factor in the estrangement.

Exploration of therapeutic space available in individual psychotherapy

These countertransference reactions, as they may be named, are interesting to note and lead to the question of whether the author is able to show unconditional love towards her patients and, if so, whether this would be desirable. Similarly to what we know of most research about general counselling and psychotherapy, the most transformative aspect of individual therapy for people experiencing family estrangement is also the quality of the therapeutic relationship. 'In describing their therapist as being a kind and compassionate person, some (in one study) went on to identify their therapist as being loving and nurturing, acting as a substitute or surrogate parent' (Blake, Bland & Imrie, Accepted/In press).

In the experience of the author, clients attending individual psychotherapy often feel it is difficult to make changes (both psychological and practical) without the security of family relationships as they feel emotionally fragile and insecure. If patients don't trust the therapist much of what is said can be perceived as an attack. It is a risk for a patient to allow their therapist into their fragile world that has taken much to stabilise and still feels vulnerable to any criticism. All decisions can feel like the wrong one: the choice to estrange as well as attempts to reconcile. It sometimes feels nearly impossible to make the right decision without any regrets. Perhaps this is just how it is to be human. But perhaps there is something particular to note for people estranged from those closest to them.

Estrangement can be freeing as it allows people who have struggled for a long time to step away from damaging relationships and to make the choice to live in a different way. It can be difficult, however, to go forwards without ever looking back or to be able to shed the old skin fully. Therapy potentially offers a space free from judgement, taboo or agenda where difficult and conflicting feelings can be fully explored. Clearly for this to be possible it would depend at least in part upon the counter-transference and/or biases, whether conscious or unconscious, of the therapist.

Reflecting on her own private psychotherapy practice, the author notes some of the clouds that overhang the therapeutic space. Estrangement brings into the light one of our most primal fears: the irredeemable loss of a child or parent. At the same time one can live vicariously through one's patients, imagining cutting off the family members that cause most irritation or hurt albeit without having to experience the personal heartbreak that this cutting off also brings.

In working with one patient in his forties, who is estranged from his father and considering estrangement from his mother, the main feelings evoked in the author, the therapist in this instance, were deep sadness and intense frustration. Sadness that this patient has not experienced unconditional love from either parent, and frustration that despite being rejected again and again, regardless of his attempts to be loving and giving, he does not walk away from the relationship, and neither does his mother recognise his continued commitment to her.

This patient has made the decision to be estranged from his father and this is extremely painful although he feels clear that he is better off without the pressure of this relationship on him. It seems that rather than unconditional love being a promise to love no matter what, it can become a pressure to bear beyond what is fair or reasonable. The loving can become very one-sided. If we see it as the parent's role to help their child to grow up and individuate, then, without the unconditional love that is required for a 'secure base' (as described by Bowlby, 1988) to be developed, is the contract of the relationship broken? Should children be free from the pressure to love their parents unconditionally?

In terms of countertransference in this therapist-patient relationship it could be considered that frustration felt by the author is a projection of her own desire to be free of parents who have not enabled her to develop a guilt-free separate self. What possibilities for this patient might be closed down by her own desire for freedom from pressure and guilt? Can she love her patients free from any agenda for them, free of memory and desire, (Bion, 1967)?

Unconditional love for therapy patients

Returning to the question of whether the therapist can and should love their patients unconditionally, two ideas are brought to mind. The Rogerian notion of unconditional positive regard, a key component of the therapeutic relationship, and Freud's idea that 'psychoanalysis in essence is a cure through love' (McGuire, 1974).

Winnicott (1960) draws out the parallels between therapy and parenting. It could be seen that there is a parallel between the therapeutic relationship that, from the beginning, is always leading to its own dissolution, and parenting, which could be designated successful when it leads to a healthy separation between parents and grown children. Although the two relationships look quite different it is clear that there are some similar functions. The love in therapy is, however, relatively explicit about its conditions from the outset and expects little love in return. Eventual estrangement is inevitable and indeed expected.

Unconditional love could be viewed through the lens of the Lacanian idea of our unconscious desire to return to a merging with the mother where all our needs and desires are satisfied. Zizek argues from the Lacanian idea that 'the moment we enter the symbolic order, the immediacy of the pre-symbolic Real is lost forever, the true object of desire ("mother") becomes impossible/unattainable' (Zizek, 1996). To develop consciousness and become a separate self requires an acceptance of our own lack and the lack in others. The implications of this for love between family members is significant. Perhaps one consequence of our separateness and uniqueness as individuals is that we cannot also have the unconditional love of our infant selves or of fantasy. We might prefer to believe in the utopian ideal that perfect and unconditional love exists rather than accept our own lack, in this case maybe the pain of our own aggression, selfishness and jealousy, and have to work through conditional and less than perfect relationships.

But this is perhaps conflating unconditional with perfect love. This is surely a standard too high even for love between parent and infant let alone between adults. Can unconditional love exist that respects the autonomy and desires of both family members whilst also accepting that mistakes will be made by all? If the parent has successfully raised a child who is an autonomous individual who chooses to cut themselves off from a relationship that they experience as painful or limiting, can an unconditionally loving parent accept this choice even if they are hurt in the process? This suffering appears to be squarely within the meaning of agape even if this aspect of unconditional love may have been lost to a modern society. This seems to reflect the idea that a human who rejects God's supposedly unconditional love is condemned to hell – definitions of which include anything from separation from God to eternal punishment. Perhaps these notions give some indication of the anger and rejection a parent whose child has estranged themselves may feel. Love is complicated and perhaps unconditional love only wishful thinking.

Disclosure statement

No potential conflict of interest was reported by the author.

References

Agllias, K. (2017). *Family estrangement, A matter of perspective*. London: Routledge.

Bion, W. (1967). Notes on memory and desire. *The Psychoanalytic Forum*, *2*(3), 279–80.

Blake, L., Bland, B., & Imrie, S. (Accepted/In press). The counselling experiences of individuals who are estranged from a family member. *Family Relations*, 1–28.

Bowlby, J. (1988). *A secure base: parent-child attachment and healthy human development*. London: Reoutledge.

Lacan, J. Seminar XII, 23rd June, (1965).

Lebey, B. (2001). *Family estrangements: How they begin, how to mend them, how to cope with them*. Atlanta: Longstreet Press.

McGuire, W. (Ed). (1974). *The correspondence between Sigmund Freud and C. G. Jung (1906–1914)*. Princeton, NJ: Princeton University Press. Retrieved from https://zizek.livejournal.com/2266.html

Winnicott, D. (1960). The theory of the parent-infant relationship. *International Journal of Psycho-Analysis*, *41*, 585–595.

Zizek, S. (1996). 'From desire to drive: Why Lacan is not Lacaniano'. *Atlántica de Las Artes 14 Otoño*. https://zizek.livejournal.com/2266.html

Romance and murder

Sally Parsloe

ABSTRACT

Bettelheim's 'The Uses of Enchantment' describes the way in which inner conflicts are processed by children in the symbolism and fantasy of fairy tales. In this paper, the author suggests that romance may be used as an adult form of fairy story and possess the same function, which is to allow prohibited desires and past trauma to be processed. Romance can be a fantasy in which essential images of the self are sustained and the past re-worked. Romance, therefore, demands the creation of a reflective image, draped over the other, like a costume. Collusion and complimentarity, as described by R.D. Laing, are required to maintain the fantasy. However, when the image threatens to have a life of its own, defences are activated, counterdefence ensues, and romance may become murderous. The ideas of Bettelheim, Freud, Klein and Laing are referred to, and a case study presented of the experience of a client whose romance has turned to murderousness.

The author works as a therapist but also as a Family Law Solicitor and a Family Mediator. She has been working with people experiencing relationship breakdown for 30 years and seen hundreds of cases professionally, as well as taking an interest in relationships around her and experiencing her own relationships.

In the work, some people come because it is 'all over', some come while the relationship is on-going but 'in trouble', some come at the beginning of a relationship, and some come for what they call 'a yearly MOT'*.

The thoughts that follow arise from the author's observation that people who were once partners in romantic love often end up feeling as if they are being killed by each other. Why does romantic love turn in some cases to murderous feelings?

It might be helpful when working with clients to think about romance as a continuation of the psychic family romance initially articulated by Freud, and developed by those who followed. In Freud's Oedipal romance, the young child is desperately in love with mother or father. Terrifying sanctions for this love lurk, the fear of castration or dreadful parental retribution. The successful navigation of the Oedipus Complex involves resignation to the prohibition that Mother and Father are not available for sexual love and the consolation that one day, the permitted prince or princess will come. The figure of the prince/princess, of the desired father and wicked step-mother, of the child in jeopardy, abandoned and wandering, of dragon slaying and winning the fair maiden, of being awoken by a kiss, are constants in fairy stories. As Bettelheim says, (Bettelheim 1976, p. 115) the fairy story has unequalled value in helping the child with Oedipal conflicts. In this symbolic land, in phantasy, desire and disappointment, abandonment and cleaving, identity and value can be worked through and understood without actually having to slay dragons.

The latency period affords a time for desire to go to sleep and dream. Erotic desire flows underground. Awaking, the object of desire and the aim of desire have emerged (all being well) to be felt as directed to the permissible, not the parent. That, of course, could also be seen as a fairy story. All is not what it seems to be. The permissible and the parent may not be so separate, nor the notion of child/adult duality. The separations are as much a figment of the imagination as dragons and witches, but the adult and the child in the adult is deprived of the fairy tales that beckon towards understanding and reconciliation. What do children do when deprived of the mirroring object of their love in which they can experiment with their reflections? One thing may be to create a substitute out of whatever is available. Romance, while it may have positive purposes and outcomes, may be also used as an adult substitute for fairy stories.

In Freud's saga, the relational conflict may be satisfactorily resolved, the circle closed, once the child accepts the difference between what is permissible and what is not. The Freudian child slays the dragon of desire, and claims the beautiful princess (to be collected sometime in the future). In fairy stories we never hear what happens afterwards beyond the epitaph that 'They all lived happily ever after'.

A more terrifying version of the Freudian family romance came from Melanie Klein. Her ideas of the horror of babyhood are the true darkness of fairy stories. There is no Walt Disney for Kleinians.

In the story of Snow White, the huntsman is told by the wicked step - mother to take Snow White into the wood and kill her, not just to kill the child, but to bring back her heart and lungs so that step-mother may eat them. In my work with people whose romances have crumbled it sometimes feels as if they want to cut out and eat each other's hearts.

We make an attempt at understanding and negotiating ourselves as desiring creatures in the world at age three to five, but we need to do it again, as adult desire emerges. The name adults give to the fantasy land in which they sometimes continue to attempt to come to terms with the power and complexity of their desire is romance. Romance is one of the few areas of socially sanctioned expressions of excess of passion, a means of acting out looked on indulgently, encouraged by the constant images in media and advertising that stimulate the creation of an object enabled fantasy that love is safe, confirming, unconditional, and unthreatening. The multi-million-pound industry that is Mills and Boon** provides formatted instructions for its authors that the heroine must fall in love despite herself, that she must navigate a dilemma, that the loved one teaches her a lesson about herself, and that once she submits, she may live happily ever after, a return to pre-symbolic semiotic bliss.

Commercial romance, however, is a castrated form of the fairy tale. There are only shades of pink velvet, no black unending forest, which is the landscape of the immense wilderness of the Post-Romantic era.

The object of adult romantic desire, now no longer mother or father but the long promised permissible substitute, bears an uncanny trace of mother or father under the mask of youth and beauty. We deceive ourselves that that trace is in our imagination, so that we can enter, by means of self-deception, the convolution of at long last possessing the prohibited, masquerading as the permitted. We want it, but we know it is prohibited. We contort, distort, deny, squint sideways and don't look in order not to acknowledge we are trying to have our cake and eat it, to love mother and to kill her, to love her purely and to make love to her, to steal father from mother and have his babies, as the case may be. In fairy tales, as Bettelheim points out (Bettelheim, 1976, p. 115), the child can have the best of both worlds. In fantasy, a girl can win out over the wicked witch (her mother) and a boy can slay the dragon (his father) while retaining (in reality) the mother and father for care and protection. In *The Splitting of the Ego in Defence Processes* (1938) Freud talks about the crafty way in which the ego manages to grant to the id its conflicting desires, and of the consequent cost to the ego of this duplicity, being the formulation of a rift, or split in the ego, for as Freud points out, nothing in life is free.

In the Kleinian lexicon, the infant's terror of abandonment by mother gives rise to murderous rage with that very same abandoning love object, such storms of feeling managed by splitting, good breast versus the monster of the oral sadistic breast, two completely different entities in the eyes and mouth of the tiny baby, who has no idea that the lovely warm milky mother is also the one who leaves him howling and alone. In the heady days of early romance, in the words of the song, '*When a man loves a woman, if she's bad he can't see it, she can do no wrong, loving eyes can't ever see*' (Lewis and Wright, 1966).

Just as the baby's state of helplessness makes him vulnerable to the unmanageable power of his own emotion, so too does the state of being helplessly in love. In love, we have the same ravenous desire for exclusivity and permanent merger.

We place impossible demands on the other, we want to be endlessly fed, to be soothed and elated, we invest the romantic object with endless goodness, and just as the baby feels hopeless despair when mother goes away, so do we when the romantic object inevitably (meta-psychically and physically) goes away. At this point we are called upon to recalibrate expectation in the face of reality.

Here the romantic endeavour comes to a watershed, having the potential to turn into what some might call mature love, or to become overwhelmed with rage and feelings of betrayal and loss, echoing the parallel between Klein's paranoid schizoid position (romance) and the depressive position (mature love).

Why do some romances seem (and all is seldom what it seems in fairy tales or in romance) satisfactorily to be able to navigate this painful eye -opening transition into mutual relationship with another person, and some don't?

One field of possibility is in what happens in the contiguity of the structures of the individuals' respective defence mechanisms and the nature of what it is that each defends (nothing less than the essential image of the self), with the latter determining in the experiences of infancy the shape of the former. We need relationships with others to work out our own identity, but those relationships can also shatter and impede the recognition of our identity. As Laing puts it 'Every relationship implies a definition of self by other and other by self.' (Laing, 1961, p. 69) A child's identity is formed in the crucible of the parental relationship. Later adult relationships are entered, through which a person may develop understanding of his identity, or fantasies of his identity. The latter requires a complicated network of reflecting and interlocking collusions, which dynamic can result in guilt and shame (Laing, 1961, p. 93.) In romance, we find the character of the handsome prince, and his inevitable corollary, the beautiful princess. The characters cannot exist alone. They need and make each other. So, if the prince turns out on closer inspection to be not so handsome, what does it mean for the beautiful princess? One meaning is that she is not so beautiful, and thus for the princess who wishes to retain her fantasy of beauty, it is necessary to maintain the handsomeness of the prince by averting her eyes from imperfection and further, to imbue the prince with a handsomeness he never had, perhaps never wanted and which feels 'not himself'. He understands however that it is required of him to be handsome and feels bad if he isn't. He cannot escape the prison of the requirement of handsomeness, even though he knows he isn't handsome. He lives in fear of his non-handsomeness being revealed, so he adopts a handsomeness he doesn't want and is then blamed for pretending to be something he isn't *and* for not being what he is pretending to be. He sustains the princess' fantasy of herself through her fantasy of him, and it is enough to drive him mad. He no longer trusts his own feelings or sense of reality. This is a major simplification of the relational trouble Laing describes in speaking of deception, collusion and complementarity in *Self and Others*.

In the desire for and fantasy of unconditional one-ness with endless good (the starting point of many a romantic relationship), defences are lulled. What is defended is exposed. Early experiences of attack, of disappointment and deception, rage and fear, consigned to the unconscious, are agitated.

The experience of being attacked is doubly shocking to the lover because it comes from the idealised object of desire, who is now no longer only within, as in the fantasy merger, the internalisation of the desired person, (indeed the created desired person who will reflect the created desired self) but who is now also outside and with a life of its own, separate and hostile. Defensive retaliation is swift and sure. The soldiers of defence (inter alia, denial, displacement, projection, splitting) awake with a shock and mobilise. Defensive counter-attack is launched on that which is defended in the other, that is, the other's signature vulnerability, engendering counter-counter attack. Battle intensifies. Unforgivable wounds are inflicted. The ideal, which has been held as but is not and never has been the other, but a field of facilitation of the unknown desires of self and other, locked in endless reflection, in threatening to have a life of its own, causes recollection, resentment and fear. In order to preserve the ideal, the other's (and consequently our own) life of its own has to be killed.

Let me cite an example from the room which shows what can happen when vulnerabilities collide.

A man went to therapy because he was having an affair and the affair was going badly. He said everything was falling apart. He no longer knew what he thought or felt or whether he was even himself, if there had ever been such a thing as himself.

He had been married over twenty years, with children, but had fallen powerfully in love with a woman that his wife had introduced him to. The affair had been going on for five years. His wife and his lover were two completely different types of women, he said. When he first met her, his lover was 'out in the world', an accomplished musician and a member of a highly regarded orchestra, funny, independent and self-possessed. She was sexually confident, which he was not (he had been impotent with his wife for many years). For the first few years of the relationship they had never argued. He could not bear to be without his lover. She existed in the forefront of his mind all the time. He could talk to her about deep feelings, which he had never done with his wife, they played well together, and sex was great. She was tender and encouraging with him, and very loving. She made him feel whole, alive, potent and part of the world again.

But that had changed and now she could at times be so angry with him that he was really frightened of her.

His wife, 'on the other hand' was a 'good' woman, and a pillar of the community. She had never worked, but did good works in the locale, looked after the family, and provided his children with a 'Rolls Royce' mothering service. He had never seen her nasty to anyone, she never did anything hurtful, she was not a liar. However, ten years into the marriage and after two children, he said he had become a fat, lonely, depressed alcoholic.

His wife, who had known of his growing relationship, saw his affair as a bitter betrayal but did not leave or ask him to leave. She burned with silent resentment that he had 'brought her into disrepute' in the community and in the eyes of the children, though it was she who told her friends and the children about the affair. His children and friends disapproved strongly. He felt saturated in guilt for the shame he was bringing to the family.

He thought now there was something mentally wrong with his lover, she got so angry and levelled horrible accusations about his wife which were not true. He even wondered if she was psychotic and he described her as abusive to him. He felt that his lover was making him ill but he still found it unbearable when they had periods when she cut off contact with him and he longed for her body, particularly her breasts.

The client had a longing, strangely romantic view and way of speaking of his own mother, whom he still called Mummy. Smiling with indulgence and love, he described her golden hair and beautiful face and curvy figure. However, after he had been in therapy for three years, he suddenly said, to the surprise of the therapist, 'My mother shagged a man on the floor. I saw them through the window.' The client was seven at this time. His father had discovered the affair but no one ever spoke of it in family, and now it was as if it never happened. There had also been an incestuous sexual relationship in the immediate family, which had never been discussed after the immediate revelation by an aunt, and which the client referred to as 'just in the imagination, something that nobody really thought had happened'. When I wondered what his mother's affair might have been like for his father the client said 'humiliating' When I wondered what it might have been like for him he said aggressively 'I haven't got a problem with my mum. I was her little man.' However sometimes great blobs of anger with his mother reared up only to be closed down immediately. The client had a club foot, and one day he shouted 'If my mummy hadn't smoked while she was pregnant, maybe my foot would have grown straight. But then how could she have known, in those days?' His anger with his mother was always rescinded by a statement of her goodness instantly afterwards.

The client was extremely resistant to the therapist exploring his relationship with his wife and mother. The sessions focused on the madness and badness of his lover, whom the client sometimes referred to as his mistress. When the therapist commented that that was quite an old -fashioned word, the client said 'No, she doesn't like it either. Or the other names.' It seemed that the client's wife had a derogatory language for his lover, including names like Flubberguts and Old Pussy. The client had told his lover that this was how she was designated in his family. But, the client added, one had to have sympathy for his wife. The nasty names were just because his wife was hurt and it made him feel very sorry for his wife, bringing home to him just how hurtful his affair was for her. It had not occurred to him that his relaying of these names to his lover might be hurtful to her. The therapist noticed that the client evaded any line of discourse that involved any implication that his wife might have any role in the difficulties in the marriage. What he could not stand in his mistress was when she started to attack his wife. These attacks, relayed indignantly by the client were that the client's wife was openly in love with another woman, disparaged and humiliated the client in many ways, excluded him, used him for money and as a beard for her own affair, manipulating her power over the children and their social group to control him. The lover said that the wife hated her because her relationship with the client threatened to pull off the wife's beard and expose her own long term relationship with her close female friend as being beyond friendship. The client denied that any of this was true and ascribed the lover's 'false accusations' as borne out of anger. When the therapist asked why she should feel angry, the client said he didn't know. However, it emerged that for some years the client had been saying to his lover that he would leave his wife, going into quite some detail as to how this would practically be implemented, and that he wanted a life married to his lover. In anticipation of this the lover had left her own husband with her children, which caused quite some sadness and financial hardship for her, but the client had not then left his own marriage. The client sorrowfully said that he had had to tell his lover all the unkind things his wife said about her, how his children hated and resented her, how his friends classed her as a 'scarlet woman'. He said she had been really silent and withdrawn when he told her he liked the idea of himself as a man who could 'go round and shag the mistress and then go home to his wife for dinner'. He could not see why this had seemed to upset his lover. In response he had told her that her anger was 'repellent' and was again surprised when the therapist wondered if this might be hurtful for the lover. When the therapist wondered in what way the client was abused by his lover, he said she had sent him an e mail saying she 'no longer wished to be Mummy's scapegoat'.

The client accepted that his wife had a very close female friend, whom she saw every day, with whom she went on holiday, decided all her important issues, including which schools his children went to, and who was round at the house 'all the time, curled up on the sofa cuddling'. When they went on holiday, his wife and her friend slept in the same room and he had to find any place in the villa he could to bed down. Seemingly without any sight of possible implications, the client described how his wife, with shining eyes, recounted that the first time she saw her friend, 'their eyes met across a crowded room and she knew she had met her soul mate'.

The therapist wondered if his wife's relationship with another woman might remind the client of the shame and anger that the client felt at his mother's infidelity. Underlying that shame however was the client's more taboo shame, his erotic desire for his mother. However, mother could not be done in, so that the shame and anger of the client and the shame of the mother had to be repressed so that she could continue to be idealised. 'Mummy' became a metaphor for the fusion of what was repressed and that which defined the main mechanism of the client's defences, splitting and projection. The therapist was also reminded of Freud's insight (*On the Universal Tendency to Debasement in the Sphere of Love. 1912*) as to the way in which impotence might be caused if a man cannot tolerate any convergence of his affectionate feelings and his sexual desire towards one person, erecting a barrier between the sacred and the profane. In this man's case, he could not shag his wife, as his mother had been shagged, he could only shag his mistress and then return to his wife for dinner. The two were forever split, as he had to split off the sexual side of his mother and his sensuous feeling towards his mother (profane and dangerous) to see her as golden and good (sacred and safe) and as he had to split off his desire for his wife (Mummy) to retain her as sacred, and invest the lover with the debasing epithets of the being in whom his sexual desire was centred so strongly. He had put his wife (his children's mother) on a pedestal of goodness, which she couldn't get off.

As well as his own self-deceptions, the client had to contend with his wife's self-deceptions and the deceptions of his wife against the world. These had become institutionalised, and were collusive between the client and his wife, the collusion spreading to the whole family. The client's family and friends as well as the client's own system projected the client's shame at his wife's treatment of him into the client's lover. The wife was not actually Mummy but acted as a tool of Mummy. The social group and family shunned the lover, called her horrible names, and the client himself used words to her that emphasised her illegitimate status whilst denying that that was what he was doing. When the lover protested and said she felt she was being used as a scapegoat, this was designated by the client as an outrageous attack on Mummy, inflating the badness of the lover who had to bear the punishment for being at once the symbol of the forbidden object of the client's sexual desire and the betrayal of it.

When the therapist wondered if the lover's feeling of being scapegoated might have something in it, the client refuted this and said, quite victoriously, that his lover was so difficult because of her relationship with her mother. Her mother could never be 'wrong', or 'bad' and there was a father who always supported the mother. The client said his lover realised that and she said that because of this she felt it especially painful to be used, again, as the receptacle for all the bad of good mummy. The client said that it was this experience that had made her paranoid and angry and that it explained why the lover blamed his wife for things she had not done. The therapist observed that it sounded like his lover's insight into herself had been grabbed at by the client further to exonerate his wife. The client protested loudly. 'No! That's why she kicks back at my wife, she's kicking back at her Mummy. It's her Mummy that drives her insane. Not mine.' The therapist left a long silence. After some minutes, the client said, 'That's not true, is it.'

It was a moment of realisation. For as long as he could recall, the client had been surrounded by duplicity in his family of origin, and in the stories that the family told and denials that the family maintained. In his own marriage the narrative was that Mummy had no sexuality, didn't have any sexual desires, was never hurtful, was only good, and anything that contradicted that narrative was immediately suppressed, *against the evidence of his own eyes and ears.* He was cast as the villain, but as this was killing him, reducing him to an alcoholic depressive, his affair provided the family with a receptacle outside the family into which all the bad could be projected. The client's wife held an image of herself as good. The client also held this image, and fed it, and maintained it, so that he and his wife were in collusion over her identity. They also colluded about the identity of the client's lover, breaking down the image of herself that she held in such a manner that she felt that she was being killed, or that the client, her lover, had killed something in her. The client himself experienced himself as murderous and sucked up the shame of his mother and of his wife in her belief that she was held in disrepute in the community. The client's collusion that was required for all of this, he had to deny in order to maintain the collusion. The self -deception had emptied him out, he had had to abandon himself, so that nothing could really be trusted, or believed, nothing was real, and truth was murdered along with his relationships.

Returning to the beginning, the elements of fantasy and imagination that act in fairy stories as a medium for working through the unbearable in comparative safety, is replaced in the Post-Romantic era with delusion, collusion, coercion and corrosion when the other is used to perpetuate the lies people tell about themselves and to themselves about themselves to save themselves from knowing themselves.

*MOT. UK annual safety check for motor vehicles.

** Mills and Boon. Leading publisher of romantic fiction.

Disclosure statement

No potential conflict of interest was reported by the author.

References

Bettelheim, B. (1976). *The uses of enchantment*. London: Penguin.

Freud, S. (1912). On the universal tendency to debasement in the sphere of love. Contributions to the psychology of love II. In J. Strachey (Ed and Trans.), *The standard edition of the complete psychological works of sigmund freud* (Vol. 11, pp. 177–190). London: Hogarth Press and the Institute of Psychoanalysis.

Freud, S. (1938). The splitting of the ego in defence processes. In A. Phillips (Ed.), *The freud reader* (pp. 64–68). London: Penguin.

Laing, R. D. (1961). *Self and Others*. London: Tavistock.

Lewis, C., & Wright, A. Composers: 'When a man loves a woman'. 1966

Polyamory - a romantic solution to wanderlust?

Marian O'Connor

ABSTRACT

This paper will explore what is meant by polyamory, why it is presenting more frequently in recent years in the media, on online forums and in therapy rooms, and what might be considered the benefits and drawbacks of this way of relating. Challenges for the therapist working with polyamorous clients will be explored and a composite clinical case example will be given as will an example from a recent television documentary on polyamory. Both cases will be discussed using the lens of a psychoanalytic couple psychotherapist and psychosexual therapist

Introduction

What is polyamory

Polyamory is a form of consensual non-monogamy (CNM). Unlike poly-andry (one woman with more than one man) or polygamy (one man with more than one woman), which have been established in some societies for centuries, the term polyamory was not used until the 1990's and did not enter the Oxford English Dictionary until 2006, although polyamorous relationships have probably always existed in some form. Polyamory is defined as having simultaneous close emotional and/or sexual relationships with two or more other individuals, with the consent and knowledge of all partners concerned.

Polyamorous arrangements vary. A common form is a primary relation-ship (often a couple) where each partner is emotionally and sexually involved with secondary partners. Another form is non-hierarchical – with all relationships having equal status. In the case example I give later the main unit or polycule is of three people.

Polyamory is not the same as open relationships, since love is central to the discourse of poly relationships. In fact, polyamory as responsible or consensual non-monogamy usually goes hand-in-hand with a rejection of sexual excitement as the *prime* motivation for non-monogamy, although a recent study (Duplassie & Fairbrother, 2018) suggests that sex and sexuality are important components for many people in their desire to pursue polyamory and Sheff's study (2005) suggested that this way of relating allowed the women interviewed to express more fully their sexual drives, including their bisexuality.

Responsible or ethical non-monogamy, where all the parties are aware of and share a consensus on what the non-monogamous arrangements should be, is meant to be rooted in honesty and consensus. Contracts are impor-tant in order to respect, protect and preserve the foundation of the primary relationship or relationships.

Rising interest in polyamory

Interest in the polyamory as well as other CNMs has grown in recent years and there are numerous podcasts, websites and self help books on the subject. In 2006 Oprah.com conducted an online poll with over 14,000 respondents, finding 7% of women and 14% of men were currently involved in open, non-monogamous marriages (quoted in Girard & Brownlee, 2015). In 2018 polyamory was the subject of both a mainstream BBC drama series and a BBC documentary.

The rising interest in polyamory may have been stimulated by gay culture which necessarily had to grow outside the established rules of society and explored new forms of relationships. In 2005, a study found that more than 40% of gay men had an agreement that sex outside the relationship was permissible, (Guardian, 2016). In a 2004 study of 217 bisexual men and women who had sought mental health services 33% were found to be involved in some form of a non-monogamous relationship, and 54% considered this relational style to be ideal (Page, 2004).

Beck, Bonss, and Lau (2003) describe how our present society is characterised by 'reflexive modernisation' where individuals no longer have their lives set out for them or are governed by traditional social principles and expectations. As the changing economic situation has meant that traditional routes to job stability, buying a house, are no longer open to many young people, both men and women are exploring different ways of working and also of living together and apart, (Ruspini, 2014). Young people are engaged in constant 'social reflexivity' (idem,p 12), faced with choices about how to live their lives and how to establish their identity. Kimmel and Aronson (2016) write about ways in which the body and sexuality are central to this questioning and exploration.

In addition, the World Wide Web (WWW) has created opportunities to connect with like-minded others, enabling those who question or feel excluded from the norms of society to form communities which validate and foster their interests. Polyamorous individuals can now find validation, support and connection through online communities and dating apps.

The appeal of polyamory

Polyamory actively questions monogamy as the only legally and religiously sanctioned way to conduct adult intimate relationships. The privileged position of monogamy in Western culture has remained even though, in our current society, monogamous relationships are under strain. They no longer offer the certainty of long-term economic and emotional stability – 42% of marriages, gay and straight, end in divorce. Also, as connections with local communities and the extended family have lessened, there has been an increased expectation that the monogamous partnership should provide friendship, intimacy, sexual excitement, emotional stability, child care and economic security (Cherlin, 2007). At the same time, research (Finkel, Hui, Carswell, & Larson, 2014) shows that spouses are spending less time alone together and are investing less in the relationship than fifty years ago. The time couples do spend alone together can be spent with each partner on a separate laptop connecting with others via gaming or social media. As a result, over time, many people are becoming less satisfied with their monogamous partnerships.

Very importantly, there is a high rate of infidelity among monogamous couples. Secret non-monogamy or affairs differ from consensual non-monogamy in that their disclosure can lead to a sense of betrayal and desperate insecurity or to divorce and the economic and emotional distress this brings. Barker and Langdridge (2010) have concluded, 'It is within this context of searches for "new" ways of relating, and questioning whether conventional monogamy is really monogamous that attention has turned to consensual non-monogamies' (p. 754).

Whereas polyamory was once isolating and nameless, it now offers a sense of community through online forums and meetings. it brings honesty and clear boundaries into intimate relationships and it allows the heady feeling of falling to love and making new connections to be repeated rather than being consigned to happen in secret or remain as a once in a lifetime experience.

Polyamory can help avoid the trauma of divorce in couples like Heidi and Jerry who appeared in the recent BBC documentary and whom I will discuss again later in this paper. Heidi reported feeling dissatisfied and depressed in her marriage to Jerry but for the last nine years she has been in a polyamorous relationship with Joe and says she is now happy and fulfilled in her life. Jerry and Heidi did not appear to be on the verge of divorce and are able to keep together a stable family unit for themselves and their daughter.

Polyamory forces individuals to put effort into all their relationships through conversations about boundaries and timetabling rather than taking the relationship for granted. It puts less strain on each partner to be everything for the other.

Interestingly, as a couple and psychosexual therapist, many of the rules which polyamorous partnerships enforce are ones which would be beneficial to all relationship and which I might suggest to some monogamous couples. Some of these rules are around openness and honesty, discussing preferences, putting in effort and commitment into ensuring quality time together, timetabling sex.

I have found that many monogamous couples rile at the lack of spontaneity which such rules demand, even if the alternative is no sex for a year and no deep conversation for at least as long. Some clients are horrified when I suggest they timetable two or three sessions at home each week to do together the psychosexual exercises I set: one partner may claim he or she can't do mornings because of the gym; the other goes to the gym in the evening; at weekends there is cycling or football or yoga or mum and dad or friends and catching up on Facebook; the overwhelming demands of work are omnipresent. And these may be young couples, both gay and straight, without children!

Difficulties with polyamory

Polyamory can be time consuming with the timetabling and discussions involved – the rise in polyamory has been equated with the availability of the Google calendar. There are advantages in being able to take our intimate relationships for granted at times and to release time and energy for raising children, extra study, creative pursuits. Polyamory may even stymy expressions of spontaneity with a loved one when the amorous couple realise that one of them is committed to spending that time with another lover or intimate partner.

Polyamory may lead to jealousy and a feeling of being left out and inadequate for those who experience that, in their particular polycule, they are the one no one is particularly interested in. This feeling of being left out can be exacerbated in partnerships where one partner declares they want to explore polyamory while the other isn't happy with it. The language of polyamory with phrases such as 'ethical non-monogamy' and 'compersion' (experiencing joy and happiness because your partner has found joy and happiness with another) may feel confusing and even cruel to vulnerable partners who actually feel betrayed and jealous but are told for example, 'Some people find it hard to experience compersion, but it is a skill that can be learned' (Beth, 2019).

Although individuals may gain validation, information and even partners through the ever growing number of online polyamory support groups (1.25 million Google search results in May 2019), Heather Wood (2011), writing about the use of illegal online pornography, has pointed out that the seductive power of the internet can fuel a sense of omnipotence and denial of reality in vulnerable individuals, leading to compulsive and destructive behaviour. The rising interest in polyamory coincides with the rise in internet usage: is it possible that some individuals who, because of difficult early emotional experiences, feel incapable of really connecting to another, are accessing polyamory websites that give them a false sense of power and control and so avoid looking at and working through early trauma?

Henrich and Trawinski (2016) have written about the social and therapeutic challenges facing polyamorous clients. In their small study of twelve participants, nine reported struggling with experiences of marginalization directly associated with their polyamorous lifestyles. Some reported how disapproval by family and friends meant there was little emotional support for them after a painful break-up or loss. Several reported that the fear of being ostracized by society led them to resort to secrecy and lies in the outside world, however open they might be in their poly community.

Polyamorous clients may bring this struggle to therapy: Weitzman (2006) found that 38% of that population who were seeing a therapist chose not to mention that they were polyamorous to their therapist. Half of Henrich and Trawinski's (2016) respondents reported dissatisfactory or negative experiences while working with conventional therapists. A review of thirty years of studies on sexual communication showed that therapists as well as health care professionals find it hard to address their patient's sexuality (Byers, 2011) and prefer to wait until the patient or client choses to speak about it. Poly clients may not want to talk about their sexuality as they have come to talk about problems at work or a recent bereavement and are worried that talking about their romantic relationships will distract or overwhelm the therapist.

Secrecy on the part of the client may cause problems in diagnosis as one of the ways therapists get to know their clients is through building a relationship with them and having a felt sense of a connection, which will include transference and countertransference reactions. If a client is unwilling to reveal their true self, perhaps for very good reason if they believe the therapist is hostile to the concept of non-monogamy, the therapist may experience the client as dissociative, incapable of relating, narcissistic.

Challenges for the therapist

It can be problematic when therapists are confronted with clients who seek relationship help when the relationship challenges our training and conventions about what a healthy relationship should be.

As a psychoanalytic couple therapist I see the adult couple relationship as most closely mirroring the early mother/infant dyad (Morgan, 2018; Pincus, 1960), In a good enough environment, an infant will grow up to believe in the idea of a loving other who will survive being both hated and loved (Klein, 1946). Where there was a lack of early containment (Bion, 1963) the infant will grow up with a different blueprint, perhaps learning to be distrustful of relationships, fearing abandonment or suffocation (the claustro-agoraphobic dilemma as described by Rey, 1979) and will erect unconscious defences to protect itself from truly knowing another or truly knowing themselves in both their love and hate, their positive and destructive aspects.

In this context, the psychoanalytic couple therapist might view polyamory as a pathological avoidance of intimacy or perhaps as a manifestation of excessive splitting (Klein, idem) or a narcissistic personality disorder where there is a rigid need to be admired and in control in relationships and a lack of real concern for the other. On the other hand, polyamory might be viewed as a successful solution to the claustro-agrophobic dilemma, or even as a creative and playful exploration of intimacy with potential for psychological growth.

I would argue that our task as psychotherapists is not to be judgemental or over enthusiastic about our clients relationship choices. Our task is to offer a psychological container where the client or clients have the space to explore and question and where we are available to listen to our counter-transference reactions as clues to the client's internal world.

It is important that we are educated and informed about different patterns of relationships so that our shock at the revelation of diverse intimacies does not mean we close our eyes and ears to the clients experience or our experience of them in the therapy room. Girard and Brownlee (2015) point out that, despite the growing emergence of alternatives to traditional dyadic relationships, there is a lack of literature to guide therapists' understanding of how non-monogamous relationships work, what themes and common issues should be addressed and how to appropriately manage their own personal beliefs about this alternative lifestyle choice. They believe that there is vital need for training and assessment tools to be available for couple therapists as these relationships present more frequently in therapy.

Being informed means that, if we feel a sense of shock or disgust when our client talks to us, we are able to distinguish whether the shock belongs to us because of our own ignorance, naivety or personal history, or whether the shock and horror is something which is being projected by the clients and gives us information about his or her internal world. Awareness of the social and cultural reality of our clients' experiences in the world outside means that we will not necessarily be derailed by their resistance to exploring their relationships in the therapy room. Poly clients who have had to defend and protect their relationship choice among family and friends may well be defensive in therapy when there is an attempt to explore with them how they see themselves in their intimate relationships. It may be appropriate for such clients to keep their defences up until they feel safe and trusting enough to explore further. Bion advises the analyst to patiently wait *'without 'irritable reaching after fact and reason' until such time as 'a pattern 'evolves.'* (1970, p. 124).

Inevitably the therapists training and belief system and perhaps life experiences will affect what pattern we see emerging. Although a number of recent research papers suggest that those who partake in CNM have similar psychological well-being and relationship quality as monogamists (Rubel & Bogaert, 2015), I believe that many psychotherapists would question the findings in Rubel's paper. As I have already referenced, psychoanalytical couple psychotherapists are trained to see the adult couple relationship as the inheritor of patterns laid down in the early mother/infant dyad, so an intimate adult triad or quartet might inevitably be viewed as problematic.

Just as young people today are questioning established expectations and institutions, will a new generation of psychoanalytic couple therapists begin to question the teachings of Klein and the Object Relations School (Gomez, 1997) and will those wedded to attachment theory (Bowlby, 1969) question its teachings? Perhaps they will start to question the supremacy of the early dyadic relationship. In some communities communal childcare arrangements have existed for centuries and, of course, twins experience a triad from birth. Recent technological advances mean that we are seeing children of lesbian parents who were born from one mother's womb using the egg from another, and children conceived from a mix of their gay fathers' sperm and the egg from a surrogate.

It was only in 1973 that the American Psychiatric Association removed homosexuality from its Diagnostic and Statistical Manual of Mental Disorders. Most psychotherapists seeing gay couples today are interested in the quality of the relationship and would not attempt to pathologise the object choice. Will this eventually be the case for therapists working with polyamorous clients?

Case studies

1. Michael and Clara

I will discuss briefly Michael and Clara, a couple who sought therapy after the breakdown of the polyamorous relationship they had had for 15 years with Dave. Dave left the triad for a monogamous relationship with Farouk whom he had been seeing for a couple of years as part of the mutual agreement that he, Michael and Clara could seek romance with others.

The threesome had a daughter, Kia, 7, who was conceived using a mix of Dave and Michael's sperm. When Dave left he insisted, against the wishes of Clara and Michael, that Kia take a paternity test, The child was found to be biologically Dave's and he remains involved in Kia's life but less so, as his new partner feels unhappy about his continuing involvement with the family.

Michael and Clara came to see me in a state of grief and confusion. They were mourning the loss of Dave but were getting little support from family and friends who 'knew this would happen one day' and that 'they only had themselves to blame for the situation.' They missed Dave as a friend, lover, confidante and, having to reframe their relationship as a dyad rather than a triad, brought up hitherto repressed resentments. For them, the triad had given them a sense of space whereas in successful dyadic relationships the space has to be more of a psychological space: me, you, us, where each can stand back and observe the other and the self and the relationship.

Perhaps polyamory had been for Michael and Clara an attempt to resolve an early failure to mourn, to let go of the omnipotence associated with what Melanie Klein calls the paranoid schizoid stage of development and to move onto the more mature depressive position which involves a capacity to mourn, to accept the reality of self and other in their negative as well as positive aspects.

Certainly many young people are reporting that their involvement in polyamorous relationships is a transitional stage, helping them to develop a more mature, realistic view of intimate relationships where they no longer expect the other to be everything for them.

For Michael and Clara, their polyamorous relationship with Michael had enabled a phantasy where they were all of one mind where love and discussion and agreement prevailed. Conflict, anger and hate had been split off and projected into the 'misunderstanding' world outside and, more recently, into Farouk as the malevolent other.

The distress that Michael and Clara were now feeling was not caused by their being in a polygamous relationship; their distress was caused by an awakening to reality and to unacknowledged mourning and anger and hate. In many ways they presented like an individual client who comes to therapy in a similar state of confusion and anguish when, after years of an 'idyllic' monogamous partnership or marriage where disagreements and difference were not allowed, their partner has left following a secret affair.

The difference here was that, whereas family and friends might support the individual whose partner had so 'cruelly' abandoned them, Clara and Michael were without this wider support.

Michael and Clara did have one another and, albeit depleted, a version of the family they had created together. The couple did survive the trauma of Dave's leaving and in the containment of therapy they slowly started to explore letting go the false-self mask they had presented to the world and to themselves to become more real and three-dimensional in their approach to one another and to the world. They used the triangular space of couple therapy to reinforce an internal triangular space where they were able to think about their own myriad emotions and to think about their relationships with others in a more mature, less idealised way. They rekindled their sexual connection and remained committed to exploring polyamory.

2. Heidi and Jerry

In the BBC documentary on Polyamory to which I referred earlier in this paper, Louis Theroux (2018) interviewed a polyamorous couple where the wife, Heidi, was in a long-term relationship with Joe whereas her husband, Jerry, had had no relationships outside of the marriage. Heidi insisted everyone was happy with the situation and Jerry acquiesced, although his tone of voice and body language suggested he felt lonely, helpless and sad.

As I watched the programme I, in common with many viewers, felt anger and outrage at Heidi's apparent selfishness and bullying demeanour. Later, I wondered whether, in my anger and outrage, I was picking up what had been split off and denied by Jerry. Heidi had described how, before meeting Joe, she had felt depressed and trapped in her marriage; she may well have felt angered and frustrated by Jerry's passivity and masochism. Perhaps theirs had been a deeply unhappy, sado-masochistic relationship and polyamory had helped the couple to stay together and, to some degree, to grow as individuals. Heidi's aggression is tempered by gratitude, Jerry's masochism is tempered by the powerful feeling that he is being Mr Nice Guy. Their daughter seemed to appreciate the liveliness and confidence Joe brought into the house and reported getting on well with Joe's children whom she said were like brothers to her.

Technical challenges in seeing poly individuals and couples/triads

Individual therapy

If we as therapists emphasise the importance of the intimate one to one relationship in therapy, how do we work with individual clients who challenge the idea of monogamy? How would we respond if a client suggested having two individual therapists as one therapist might not provide everything the client needs?

Also, can the intimate relationship between therapist and client who is already in an intimate relationship with a partner outside therapy be seen as a polyamorous relationship? When I see couples where one partner is already seeing a therapist, I sometimes find that the individual therapist hovers like a ghost or a guardian angel in the room, protecting and guarding their client from me, the work and their partner. There can be a sense that, when I offer an interpretation or observation, the client does not engage immediately but stores the idea away for later discussion with the therapist, leaving me feeling helpless and shut out. The client's partner may report a similar feeling. This struggle to engage one of the partners in the work is similar to situations where I suspect one partner is having an ongoing secret affair.

When the 'affair' is with a therapist, the relationship is not usually a secret one and, as I have suggested, could be likened to a polyamorous relationship: one partner finds their needs are not being met by their spouse and so seeks a therapist who can fulfil particular intimacy needs. Just as in a polyamorous relationship, the spouse is expected to learn 'compersion' and feel enriched that their partner is finding enrichment in their new intimate relationship, but may end up feeling helpless and shut out. It is worth considering whether we talk enough with our individual clients about the effect of the intimate therapeutic dyad on their existing relationship/s.

Relationship therapy

Working with three or four clients coming together to discuss difficulties in their polyamorous relationship is perhaps more like group therapy than traditional relationship therapy and many couple and relationship therapists would be reluctant to take on such a case. A challenge for the therapist used to working with the centrality of the monogamous couple relationship might be to avoid trying to find what is the 'central' relationship with the other(s) being seen as satellites rather than as important to the constellation as a whole. Ritchie and Barker (2006) write that a lack such support and acceptance contributes to feelings of isolation and tension within polyamorous relationships. Henrich and Trawinski (2016) suggests that polyamorous clients can have positive and empowering therapeutic experiences with therapists who learn about polyamory and show compassionate support. In the same way the white, heterosexual and monogamous therapist might attempt to read and understand more about arranged marriages or same sex couples, perhaps it is time for non polyamorous therapists to keep an open and questioning mind when thinking about and researching polyamory.

Conclusion

This paper has been an attempt to understand why polyamory is gaining in popularity and visibility in recent years. Poly individuals, couples and triads who seek therapeutic help for their relationship may face incomprehension or disapprobation from therapists who have been raised and taught in a society which privileges monogamy. Several studies suggest that polyamorous clients may hide their polyamory from their therapists in case they are dismissed as mentally unstable. The literature suggests that therapists would benefit from wider reading and training in the field in order to offer polyamorous clients appropriate and empathetic support.

Disclosure statement

No potential conflict of interest was reported by the author.

References

Barker, M., & Langdridge, D. (2010). Whatever happened to non-monogamies? Critical reflections on recent research and theory. *Sexualities, 13*, 748–772.

Beck, U., Bonss, W., & Lau, C. (2003). The theory of reflexive modernization: Problematic, hypotheses and research programme.' *Theory, Culture and Society, 20*(2), 409–443.

Beth, L. (2019). Retrieved from: https://the-intimacy-coach.com/polyamorous-definition-polyamory-language-terms-defined/

Bion, W. R. (1963). *Elements of psycho-analysis*. London: Heinemann.

Bion, W. R. (1970). *Attention and Interpretation*. London: Tavistock.

Bowlby, J. (1969). *Attachment and loss, vol 1. Attachment*. London: Hogarth Press.

Byers, S. (2011). Beyond the birds and the bees and was it good for you?: Thirty years of research on sexual communication. *Canadian Psychology, 52*(1), 20–28.

Cherlin, A. J. (2007). The deinstitutionalization of american marriage. In S. Ferguson (Ed.), *Shifting the Center: Understanding contemporary families* (3rded., pp. 183–201). New York, NY: McGraw Hill.

Duplassie, D., & Fairbrother, N. (2018). Critical incidents that help and hinder the development and maintenance of polyamorous relationships. *Sexual and Relationship Therapy, 33*(4), 421–439.

Finkel, E. J., Hui, C. M., Carswell, K. L., & Larson, G. M. (2014). The suffocation of marriage: Climbing mount maslow with- out enough oxygen. *Psychological Inquiry, 25*, 1–41.

Girard, A., & Brownlee, A. (2015). Assessment guidelines and clinical implications for therapists working with couples in sexually open marriages. *Sexual and Relationship Therapy, 30*(4), 462–474.

Gomez, L. (1997). *An introduction to object relations*. London: Free Association Books.

Guardian (2016) Sleeping with other people: How gay men are making open relationships work. Retrieved from: https://www.theguardian.com/lifeandstyle/2016/jul/22/gay-dating-open-relationships-work-study

Henrich, R., & Trawinski, C. (2016). Social and therapeutic challenges facing polyamorous clients. *Sexual and Relationship Therapy, 31*(3), 376–390.

Kimmel, M. S., & Aronson, A. (2016). *The gendered society reader* (6th ed.). New York, NY: O.U.P.

Klein, M. (1946). Notes on some schizoid mechanisms. *The International Journal of Psycho-analysis, 27*, 99–110.

Morgan, M. (2018). *A couple state of mind*. London: Routledge.

Pincus, L. (1960). Relationships and the growth of personality. In *Marriage: Studies in emotional conflict and growth (Part I)* (pp. 11–34). London: Tavistock Institute of Marital Studies.

Rey, J. H. (1979). Schizoid phenomena in the borderline patient. In J. Le, J. Boit, & A. Capponi (Eds.), *Advances in the psychotherapy of the borderline*. New York, NY: Jason Aronson

Ritchie, A., & Barker, M. (2006). 'There aren't words for what we do or how we feel so we have to make them up': Constructing polyamorous languages in a culture of compulsory monogamy. *Sexualities, 9*, 584–601.

Rubel, A., & Bogaert, A. (2015). Consensual nonmonogamy: Psychological well-being and relationship quality correlates. *The Journal of Sex Research, 52* (9), 961–982.

Ruspini, E. (2014). *Diversity in family life; gender, relationships and social change.* Bristol: Policy Press.

Sheff, E. (2005). Polyamorous women, sexual subjectivity, and power. *Journal of Contemporary Ethnography, 34*, 251–283.

Theroux, L. (2018) https://www.bbc.co.uk/iplayer/episode/b0br9vrx/louis-theroux-altered-states-1-love-without-limits

Weitzman, G. (2006). Therapy with clients who are bisexual and polyamorous. *Journal of Bisexuality, 6*, 137–164.

Wood, H. (2011). The internet and its role in the escalation of sexually compulsive behaviour. *Psychoanalytic Psychotherapy, 25*(2), 127–142.

A phenomenology of love, thanks to Lacan, Miller, and Jellybean

Tony McSherry

ABSTRACT

This paper presents a phenomenology of love, indicating some complexities in working with the lover in psychotherapy and counselling, while taking into account Lacanian ideas about love. Experience and Lacan's ideas seem to intersect, the latter perhaps announcing a harsh 'truth' from which experience flinches. Reference to a small dog illustrates to an extent the real but illusory cause of desire we find in Lacan's object *a*. The paper begins with exploring how language can speak of the private, the phenomenological world, and therefore also says something that addresses everyone to an extent. Theory may emerge in this addressing and it can be noticed where perhaps Lacan is coming from. The lover and the broken-hearted person in therapy presents a challenge, to stay with experience or take refuge in theory, or perhaps stay with both, avoiding a collapse into technicalities. It seems that healing may begin to come through relinquishing a precious image/idea/story, of oneself, if at all possible.

Introduction – how can we speak generally of something private?

Sitting on the tube on the way here today in the stuffy air with its import of grime and grease, indeed human skin cells and engine oil, what is clear is how we are so immersed in this anonymous world of others. An anonymous world open to communication, despite the headphones, newspapers, and mobiles apparently absorbing us in such busy lives that it appears as if we must be indispensable to someone, or perhaps many others, somewhere. The living scene is as permeated with desire, uncertainties, and fantasies, as much as the air is shot through with that cloying oiliness. The young especially seem to receive a certain look, recipients of desires, of questions. Men glance interrogatively at young women, with a complex desire it seems, a kind of need that is not only lustful but sexual, as if asking questions, the most intimate ones. Miller's (2008) Lacanian assertion that we love the one who seems to harbour the answer to our question, 'Who am I?' seems to find its ground here on the underground, in the phenomenological world of being in nature and with others. Young men are perhaps more intrusive in their look but also uncertain, and old men sometimes seem to have a look of regret, and desire, something even innocent. I recall my mother giving me a bath, aged 3, and feeling accepted. Is it a similar look of affirmation and recognition these men look for, whether young or old? Do we search for a look of some affirmation of one's being in this strange other (who is a woman in this case), with remnants of sparkling infant desire and reciprocal love folded into that mother's touch and look? The 'me' seems important here, and it seems that it is the 'me' (of others) that shows itself in the briefest of glances on the underground, from all manner of men. In an uncertain relation, something of the other is found in oneself (McSherry, Loewenthal, & Cayne, 2019). It is not always only lust, and even if it is, that seems dislocated somehow from something else, a more profound experience of loss. Does love promise to cover over such a loss?

In the melee of desires, looks, jostling bodies, and personal spaces being established, I recall the anxiety of being a teenager, not knowing what is expected of me, how to be in a world shot through with desires and needs of others, what the other wants from me, while tentatively acknowledging what I want. And how does a woman show her desirous uncertainties in a world shot through with this complex look of men? Would she notice the fragility of that look, imagining instead the aggression and demand that is often real too? It is easy to begin to over-think here, and lose oneself in ideological talk in which we are already lost. If Hopkins (1970/1876-1889, p. 27) felt that the world oozed with the grandeur of his God, perhaps what he could have meant was that it oozed with the grandeur of desire, but his society could not allow such a thought. I imagine Lacan on the train reading a newspaper with the headline 'Man's desire finds its meaning in the other's desire' (Lacan, 2006, p. 222; see Fink, 1995). It points to a confusion as to whose desire is whose. After many years of exhaustive work, just as I thought I was finally thinking for myself, I catch a glimpse of myself infused with someone else's thoughts, desires, looks, whims, ideas, and so on. Staying with the bewildering confusion, the absurdity makes us pause. Lacan might call such an event a sudden awareness of the unconscious, a realisation that one's desires emanate from an enigma that shows itself under the cover of something like a surrealist painting, or a dream, that has been patched together from others' desires (see Jaanus, 1995). It seems that we are alienated in the world of others (see Lacan, 2006, p. 312) and perhaps love promises to remedy such alienation.

There seems to be something important then in the regretful looks of old men, the stuttering speech of the boy teenager, and the girl teenager looking away in embarrassment. Such indications of desire and loss seem more important than strident calls for the domination of equality. They seem to indicate something tentatively trying to speak for itself that can be easily crushed by certainties. At the risk of collapsing into certainty, Lacan's (2006, p. 222) quote above continues, to say that our 'first object(ive) is to be recognised by the other'. If this is true, how does the woman/young woman express and show her confused desires in a world dominated by the male glance? And how does the man show in his look that he is caught too in the male look even though he is looking out from it? I am suddenly in my therapy room, being a therapist to someone caught in the other's desire. Good humour, and an almost tactile care for the other seems important here, because so much is going on. It would be easy to understand too quickly, thereby missing out on an appreciation of the fabric of the psyche that is multiply layered and folded in an infinite field of meaning, coloured by feeling and the experience of strange-ness. We find the other's look in ourselves looking out.

It seems that the other's insecurity, aggression, greed, lust, violence, and so on, is only noticed because it has already found a home in our own selves. This is why Wittgenstein's (2009, PPF 327; p. 235) comment, 'If a lion could talk, we wouldn't be able to understand it,' makes sense. We can know nothing of the species of meaning whose language is established on different parameters (yet it seems too that others are a different species at times). Living as a Franciscan once, I had given away everything, all material goods including clothes and things, the money squirreled away. Yet, the small allowance we had, enough to buy a coffee twice a week in a Roman café, suddenly one day held more weight in my sleeve. A small sum loaned to a friend and not returned created and found a ground for resentment. I tried to cover the wound with a plaster of a prayer, only then to berate myself for cowardice at not facing my own avarice, and then seeing that itself as a plastering over something else. We find the trace of the other in ourselves, the acquisitive mind, the solicitous child, the vain professional, the murderer and villain. This perhaps is because we are immersed in language, that 'takes hold' of us (Lacan, 2006, p. 6). A universal language of significations permeating the sensual world (Merleau-Ponty, 1968). Don't be sentimental about it – it will kill you if you don't take it deadly seriously. This seems to be what Lacan means when, following Freud, he speaks of 'the signifier's displacement' determining 'subjects' acts, destiny, refusals, blindnesses, success, and fate, regardless ... and that everything pertaining to the psychological pregiven follows willy-nilly the signifier's train, like weapons and baggage' (Lacan, 2006, p. 21). But it seems we must find out something about this for ourselves, the phenomenological (experience) teaches us better than Lacan, just like the only way to understand the joy of a boy playing football is to be that boy. Words are forever melded into the sensual in the flying run, the stinging rain.

Speaking of love

In a similar way to trying to speak of the running boy, trying to speak of love seems impossible as it is so private. But something about the individual is made universal through the field of language, and in this way through words we can indicate something that cannot be said. The love I mean is what Zizek (2018, p. 187) calls 'authentic love ... the exclusive fixation on another being that totally derails our immersion in the rhythms of ordinary daily life'. And their lovers' talk is spoken in private sweet nothings. How can we speak of that private sweet nothing? How can the heart-broken client tell us of sweet nothing? Trying to help the broken-hearted client seems impossible, whose speech stumbles into what seems like banalities and silence.

Where does the dog, Jellybean, come in? She comes in long before the heartbreak. In a sense to think about love with someone 'in love' is like trying to think about something with the small dog. She is a mongrel, like a long-legged Jack Russell, but with black and brown fur, brindle legs, with a crooked white diamond on her chest. She loves to chase a particular thing with a fevered intensity, that thing being the contrast between light and shadow if that difference moves, careering across sofas, under cushions, behind flower pots, in a frantic drive to catch the thing she sees. I'm not sure what she sees, but what she chases seems to be defined by light and shadow, the two inseparable, one not perceptible without the other. I try to explain to her it is just a trick of the light moving, and she looks at me patiently for a moment, then struggles to be released to start the chase again. The joy in her whole being when she thinks she has caught the light/shadow thing! Her tail wagging wildly, her paws dancing on the gravel as she dives behind shrubs into the darkness. She is chasing shadows from my view, but from hers it is something real. I feel compelled to place fragments of Lacan's and Miller's thoughts on love alongside the images of Jellybean in her joyful anxiety. The thing she chases creates a boundless life-giving quest and is the obverse of the arid therapy space where joy seems to have drained from the earth when we meet a broken-hearted client. The thing she chases could be a cartoon sketch of that elusive thing, the Lacanian object *a*, the cause of desire, which is by definition outside of symbolisation or representation (Fink, 1995, p. 83). She follows its unpredictable path inexorably, her energy totally consumed by the quest despite its elusive character and how she never catches it. Talking to Jellybean about her quest is useless, as she does not have language, and as far as we know, does not speak. But talking to someone in love can make some difference if the therapist becomes the cause of desire instead. If by some magic trick, the therapist comes to be seen as object *a*, then something else might start to catch the client's eye. The magic trick is what we call transference love (Freud, 1915/1958). Otherwise, the therapist is nothing but an interested observer, a point of reference, a sounding board, maybe an encyclopaedia and information is given to the client. Instead, transference love allows for desire being put into play for the client such that his/her own desires come under question and he/she begins to wonder who they are. It seems that this aspect of the Lacanian project is like phenomenology in that it opens out towards something else that evades definition.

Speaking of one's own love is clearly wrong, because it is not only mine. It belongs to others and so it cannot be shared. But perhaps if things are turned into a kind of make-believe story at least to some extent it could belong to any love. Like Wittgenstein's lions we might understand each other. Once upon a time I was one of two creatures finding a way to negotiate the world in a cocoon of not so narcissistic self-appreciation. The cocoon was like a fragile set of shared ideals and sensuality held together by an illusory but very real sense of being. It inhabited our fingertips and very breath. If this fragile state could speak it would say something like, 'This is natural, this is what love is, and it is good.' I was always puzzled how lovers we passed by seemed to look so miserable and forlorn, as if they had read somewhere that love was meant to be tragic, and were waiting for the tragedy to hit like a half-expected avalanche. It took a while for our own avalanche to hit, and it was triggered by an ideal collapsing, exposing the ground of our individual selves as desiring something impossible. By the time we understood enough to smile and forgive each other our impossible ideals, it was too late. Some kind of material damage had been done. Love seems to vanish in the act of friendship and some other kind of love takes its place.

The feeling of an illusory ideal seems important in love, and just because something is illusory does not mean it is not real. But the repair work may take lifetimes and there are no guarantees. No wonder then in such an uncertain landscape that we are driven to attempt to bind the chimera of ideal love in a marital contract, or its equivalent, tying us up in a knot of social and financial relations, even loving ones, until 'death us do part.' If you go for a walk on Christmas day on your own, in the afternoon before it's dark, you might find this kind of love glowing out from homes, curtains pulled back, tables set, families gathered, in a weird display to those outside who walk past. The pulled-back curtains are important. They invite the outsider to look, to invoke something in the unknown stranger that is both a welcome and a rejection. You are welcome to look but you do not belong to this. It feels like there is a kind of death in the welcome and rejection of walking past. Perhaps it is an envious look that is being both invited and cast on the Christmas path, but hesitating on the road it is difficult to know who is better off, those on the inside, or what always seems to be the lone person on the outside. Love is a bit like this. It offers a welcome, an enfolding in the other that is illusory and healing, warming and stifling. It is real. Yet it seems there is something unreal about it, like Jellybean's object that draws her along. What are we encouraging when we even unwittingly encourage a client to believe they have lost something that is easy to understand when love is lost? Or that they can get it back? As therapists what kind of service are we offering if we don't know the ruins of our own love? Are we unconsciously (or not) just leading others up our own garden path? How do we respond to Lacan's challenge?

'There is absolutely no reason why we should make ourselves the guarantors of the bourgeois dream. A little more rigour and firmness is demanded in our confrontation with the human condition' (Lacan, 2008, p. 373; also see Critchley, 1998, p. 76).

Nevertheless, I don't want to believe Lacan when he says there is no such thing as a sexual relationship (Fink, 1995, pp. 104–105), yet the thought snags on something, like a woollen jumper snags on a nail and it seems we must be careful to avoid something or the whole lot will unravel. The words catch on things opening up holes in old fabrics through which metaphorical moths come flying. The duo, 'I believe him/no, I don't', flicker on and off like semaphore lights on a stormy night obscured by dark unseen waves. His words have the annoying slipperiness and dream-like quality of answers to that unnerving question, 'Who am I?' The certainty appears and asserts itself like a seabird hovering, then we take our eye off it, and it has slipped away along the coastline rising and falling somewhere else over something unseen. It's hard to be certain what Lacan means. Fink's (1995) account (sketched here) indicates that he means that those of us who are neurotic men and women relate to a third term, the world of others, demands and desires, differently. By 'men' and 'women' he means those with masculine and feminine structure respectively regardless of gender. We therefore look for something in the other to 'complete' ourselves that we do not have. As infants, in becoming feminine or masculine we have to give up some of our enjoyment (jouissance) to the world (the Other) in meeting the demands of others and the desire of others. In doing this, we sacrifice something that we are forever trying to regain. Will we ever get it back? Not really.

" … it is only insofar as we alienate ourselves in the Other and enlist ourselves in support of the Other's discourse that we can share some of the jouissance circulating in the Other" (Fink, 1995, p. 99).

A limit is placed on the infant (for example, through frustration of its demands) and in its acceptance of that he/she finds a place in the world of language, speech, discourse, communication, law, and indeed, commerce. What is in play here is a fundamental and real loss. But for the feminine what has been lost orients the subject towards finding an identity and the sublime in love, while orientation for the masculine is towards the recuperation of a thing (imagined to have returned in the illusory object *a*).

As an aside from Fink's (1995) account, it is the light/shadow thing that draws Jellybean on. Its presence and absence, its movement from one place to another without being anywhere, creates what we could call desire in her. In a homologous way, lack or loss causes us to desire in Lacanian terms. It seems important then for therapy that if we wish our neurotic clients to become desiring again, that we don't offer to 'fill the space' (with theories, ideas, our own problems) but instead open up a space for lack.

I overheard some talk in the dead of night once between two lovers (from an adjacent room with plasterboard walls), speaking softly with varying intensities, their voices sometimes lifting and cresting, insisting and dying away into whispers. I felt like a perverse moth drawn irresistibly to a lethal meaning between their words (which need to be read aloud):

'Do you love me?'
'Of course, I love you'
'You love me'
'Yes, I love you'
'But how do I know you love me?'
'I'm telling you I do'
'Do you love me?'
'Yes'
'Are you sure?'
'Yes, I'm sure. But I need to sleep, I'm tired'
'Do you love me?'
'I love you!'
'How do you know you love me?'
'I know'
'You know that you love me'
'Yes'
'How would I know that you know that?'
'I have to sleep!'
'Do you love me?'

The dialogue went on in these veins, and I fell asleep to its murmuring beat. I'm not sure where it all ended, but a friend told me a television was launched from their window at the sleepier protagonist making an escape some days later.

In this recollection it is the endless questioning and uncertainty that seems so important, seems to indicate an ontological uncertainty at the heart of the experience of love. Is the demanding protagonist privy to a sense of non-relationship and attempting to cover it over with reassurances? Does marriage try to put an end to such uncertainty? Do public signs (pulled-back curtains at Christmas), and legal frameworks of affiliation and loyalty, somehow ameliorate the uncertainty lurking at the heart of love? Is one function of social norms, culture, and discourse running through social structures, that of anaesthetizing the anxiety of uncertainty in love? These questions seem exhausting to even ask, and it seems that the more they are argued through to the bitter end the more they feel exhausting and too rationalised. Is it so painful to think something like, 'I loved you once but don't love you any more', that we need a binding legal agreement to block out that thought? The anxiety of uncertainty is bound up in signatures, witnesses, papers, and ribbons. Unsuccessfully. It hurts to think this way about something as vital as love.

That there is no sexual relationship seems too uncompromising to bear. It comes across as cold and grandiose, stretching reason beyond its limits – that we are doomed to forever rummage around in despair in the entanglements of love to find some certainty, some sense of 'being in relation.' But is it not just as hard to bear the thought that the one we love no longer loves us? And it may be harder if you are the one who is loved to bear this burden of 'not loving enough'. Nobody seems to win in love.

The thoughts here were ploughed up on finding a piece of an interview with Jacques-Alain Miller (2008), conducted by Hanna Waar, uncovering bits of ideas that appeared like fragments of broken pottery. Miller is an authority on Lacan, and the interview is titled, *On 'Love'*. Two phrases especially cut through something.

"We love the one that [sic] harbours the response, or a response, to our question: 'Who am I?'" (Miller, 2008, p. 116),

"Love is a labyrinth of misunderstanding whose way out does not exist" (Miller, 2008, p. 120).

Note the word 'harbour' in that we do not offer an answer but it appears as if we have one. These phrases impinge on some complacency, like the sight of the Christmas parlours offering both a welcome and exclusion. There is something attractive when another person makes room for us, for me, not rushing away, being present, and at least trying to be available without being in a hurry. We know when this happens. It sometimes seems perverse that people have to pay us therapists for it to happen (if they're lucky). We are willing to stay in the labyrinth, walking alongside them like fellow travellers who are supposed to know (Lacan, 1978), hopefully not lazily basking in the limelight.

Being with the broken-hearted, wounded person, through endless hours of questioning and puzzling, staying patiently with the question as to why the lover no longer loves, does indeed seem like being lost in a labyrinth. Can we patiently stay with the client who chases the lost object *a*, and in the process finding something about themselves that is revelatory? Answers don't come easily, if at all, and those that come are snatched at too hastily, or not accepted. The fault is often placed in the other. A windfall of faults, skulduggeries, and even sins, is shaken out of memories mostly imagined. And not many come to admit, 'There must have been something about me they didn't like.' In other words, can I allow the other person *not* to love me? Or not to love me enough? If I can't, then what does that mean? Is it possible to say, 'It's okay, you don't have to love me that much'? It's hard to say this when you have *felt* loved by the other.

There is an endless circling around questions addressed to the other person who is no longer there. And this kind of questioning may easily end in destruction of the other's image, or of one's own image, or both. What kind of rage is released when we refuse to allow that we are not the be-all and end-all of someone else's life? Surely, questions like these are not too hard to hold onto in our minds? But in harsh reality they are, of course. It seems to be the work of the therapist to hold on to those questions, reposing them, reframing them, until something else emerges. Death might show itself.

It seems like a kind of death to allow room for something other than rage or vengeance. We have to embrace a death perhaps to do so – perhaps the death of an image of oneself. Those of us who cannot, or refuse to, let go of that rejected image surely are losing out on something. Images tend to sediment, precipitate, fossilise something living. It seems as if we hold on to something, an embodied image, that feels like an ' … 'experience" of truth" (Husserl, 1970, § 51 in Welton, 1999, p. 21). In that image words belong to a memory that has a living breath. Accepting the loss of an image that is living, a living breathing image, seems to open out something new, that may not even be perceptible at first. But it is almost pointless to say this to someone who is broken-hearted. We are asking them to die in some way. Yet, embracing this death, something shows itself again, glimpsed like a dragonfly cuts the air. We realise that somehow we are not dead. It must be a partial death then. Not a death of the self, but death of an image of the self that was covering over something new. Some other image takes its place. I am reminded of Jellybean, who starts up her quest again when the light/shadow thing reappears (inexplicably to her) in some other guise. She doesn't see that I can see the clouds clearing so new light/shadow things will start to move in the breeze. Perhaps this is one way of thinking of theory – that it enables us to see further than our clients while also bearing in mind that we know very little or nothing of their ' … ' experience" of truth" (Husserl *ibid*).

It seems also that something persists beneath the self-image that has been let go. We don't seem to shed the beloved when the image of ourselves as beloved falls away. There must be something that remains; the beloved lives all along as the beloved even if he/she is hated now, cloaked with hatred. We say things like, 'I hate you, my love', betraying the contradiction at the heart of everything.

In place of a conclusion

A dark light seems to flicker in the heart of us human beings, we who can hate the one we love. It seems that this contradiction in love must not be collapsed into technicalities – psychodynamics, intense existential views, or cognitive metalwork that would encase the mind. Lacan's work, which seems akin to a phenomenological stance, appears to open out on to new possibilities. But if you try to catch the contradiction you might break its wings, killing any possibility of redemption in relationships. Or should I say forgiveness. Forgiveness seems to come if we are able to place the precious image of ourselves to one side, like a beloved story we have grown tired of reading. Although placing the image and the story to one side breaks the heart all over again, it is broken differently now in order to be set right. Perhaps this is where Miller's (2008) word 'harbour' resonates at different levels. A harbour is a place of refuge, and where things get repaired, but it also indicates a place of intentions that come to be understood and spoken.

Acknowledgments

Thanks to Liz Nichols for her comments on an earlier draft of this paper.

Disclosure statement

No potential conflict of interest was reported by the author.

References

Critchley, S. (1998). "Das Ding": Lacan and Levinas. *Research in Phenomenology, 28,* 72–90.

Fink, B. (1995). *The Lacanian subject: Between language and Jouissance.* Princeton: Princeton University Press.

Freud, S. (1915/1958). Observations on transference-love (Further recommendations in the technique of psychoanalysis III). *Standard Edition of the Complete Psychoanalytical Works of Sigmund Freud, 12,* 157–171. London: Hogarth Press.

Hopkins, G. M. (1970/1876-1889). *Gerard Manley Hopkins: Poems and prose.* (W. H. Gardner, Ed.). Harmondsworth, England: Penguin Books.

Husserl, E. (1970). *Logical Investigations.* [Husserliana 19]. (J. N. Findlay, Trans.). London: Routledge & Kegan Paul.

Jaanus, M. (1995). The *Démontage* of the Drive. In R. Feldstein, B. Fink, & M. Jaanus (Eds.), *Reading Seminar XI: Lacan's Four Fundamental Concepts of Psychoanalysis* (119–136). New York, NY: State University of New York Press.

Lacan, J. (1978). *The four fundamental concepts of psychoanalysis.* (A. Sheridan, Trans.). Norton: New York.

Lacan, J. (2006). *Écrits, the first complete edition in English.* (B. Fink, H. Fink, & R. Grigg, Trans.). New York: W. W. Norton & Co.

Lacan, J. (2008). *The ethics of psychoanalysis 1959-1960: The seminar of Jacques Lacan, Book VII.* J-A. Miller (Ed.) (D. Porter, Trans.). London: Routledge.

McSherry, T., Loewenthal, D., & Cayne, J. (2019). A phenomenology of the therapeutic after Husserl and Merleau-Ponty. *Existential Analysis: Journal of the Society for Existential Analysis, 30.1*(Pearl Edition), 128–143.

Merleau-Ponty, M. 1968. *The Visible and the Invisible.* C. Lefort Ed. A. Lingis, Trans. Evanston: North Western University Press.

Miller, J.-A. (2008). On aime celui qui répond à notre question: □Qui suis-je?□. *Psychologies Magazine, 278*(Octobre), 116–120. English translation by Adrian Price: http://www.nlscongress2018.com

Welton, D. (1999). *The essential husserl: Basic writings in transcendental phenomenology.* Bloomington: Indiana University Press.

Wittgenstein, L. (2009). *Philosophical investigations* Revised 4th. J. Schulte & P. M. S. Hacker Eds. G. E. M. Anscombe, P. M. S. Hacker & J. Schulte, Trans. Oxford: Wiley-Blackwell.

Zizek, S. (2018). *The courage of hopelessness: Chronicles of a year of acting dangerously.* London: Penguin Books.

Conversations outside the walls of the city: Techniques, erotic love and the wings of desire in *Phaedrus* and psychotherapy

Onel Brooks

ABSTRACT

This paper about the desire to keep even ourselves under control and in order, does not set out to show that the author, having himself under control and in order, is able to make masterful links between psychoanalytic theory and practice. It is a paper that takes up and illustrates with client work Socrates' argument in Plato's dialogue, *Phaedrus*, that although technical mastery and self-control are necessary, without the madness of love and passion, what is produced and the life that is lived is limited, arid, crude, unfulfilled and unfulfilling. The paper shows a passion for speaking and listening that may help to take our conversations outside the walls of the city: outside of where we usually speak and listen, outside of 'normal', 'natural' and permitted.This passion for listening and speaking is a divine madness, that can help to lift us out of foolish, complacent and calculative ways of being, inspiring us to consider and revere another person and our own existence. Love in this dialogue is not something that we have under our control. It is rather something that might lead us to philosophy as Plato seemed to value it, to speaking about what is important to us, to companionship and conversation.

Introduction

When some clients speak about being in 'open relationships' and being 'polyamorous', they speak of agreeing to and encouraging the person they are in a relationship with to see and have sex with other people, so long as no one develops 'feelings for' or falls in love with a third person. They may even state in their agreement the frequency with which the lover is able to have sex with the lover's lover, or that pictures or videos of the lover's lover must be shown. It often seems as if they feel that they are in control of and above love and desire, as if they believe that making contracts is a way of contracting -in the sense of making smaller and more manageable- the potential chaos and madness inherent in our passions.

In this paper, I do not present myself as someone who is in control of love, desire and the potential chaos, confusion and frustration of engaging with another person. Mastery of theory and practice is not demonstrated by outlining clear links between them. The reader is invited to a conversation with a client, my conversation with myself about this series of meetings, and to a conversation about one of Plato's dialogues; there is very little in the way of explicitly applying theory in this paper. Indeed, a little reflection may help to make it clear that a paper concerned with the desire for techniques to master desire is unlikely to try to demonstrate mastery of psychoanalytic theory and technique.

Two ways of relating and speaking are contrasted in this paper. The first regards our being together and speaking as having obvious and clear purposes, as a matter of efficiency in the pursuit of advantageous ends, narrowly conceived. For the second way of being together and speaking, this first way may have its place in the courtroom, or the boardroom, the committee meeting, but it is not how friends, lovers, and other people who are intimate with each other, speak to each other. An approach to psychotherapy that is not too caught up in contracting, protocols and prescribed routes, may leave room for this second form of speaking and relating.

After an illustration of working with a client who seemed to desire to be above and in control of longing, loving and desiring, I turn to Plato's dialogue, *Phaedrus*, and in particular Socrates' claim that although technical mastery and self-control are necessary, without the madness of love and passion, what is produced is limited, arid, crude, unfulfilled and unfulfilling. I try to show that this enchanting, complex dialogue from another time and place addresses important issues that we meet inside and outside of the consulting room.

Beginning

My new client arrives for the first of her six sessions. An attractive woman in her mid-twenties, looking as if she is dressed for the beach, sits legs crossed and exposing, smiling at me. I say, 'Perhaps you could tell me why you are here?' Still smiling and looking deep into my eyes, she respond with something like, 'I don't have any problems really; well, apart from the fact that there are so many men and such little time'. Still looking deeply into my eyes, she tells me that she prefers older men; men around her age are still boys who don't quite know what they are doing. Older men have had more practice.

Rather than sit there looking into her eyes as she stares into mine, as if locked into a duel with her, I look away from her eyes, then realise that she is too uncovered for me to drop my gaze without looking away from her and at the carpet next to her. The room seems to be smaller than usual. It is as if I am backed into a corner of it. I do not know why she has come to see me and what she wants.

Something changes in me. Looked up from my refuge in the carpet, and perhaps acting out my feelings of being confronted by confronting her -

rather than trying to reflect on them- I hear myself say something like, 'It sounds like we had better begin by talking about you and your father'. She changes instantly from seductress to someone who is very angry. 'What are you talking about him for? What has he got to do with it? I hate him.' She tells me Dad is a 'bastard' who left her mother when my client was quite young. When she saw Dad later, he was full of bitterness about her mother. I heard as a curse as well as a lament, Dad's pronouncement that no man would ever really love my client's mother nor my client. Yes, they could get men to have sex with them, but no man would ever really love them. (I thought I heard her father's declaration of his love for my client's mother and my client, but a bitter declaration, the passionate utterances of a man driven mad by something. What though? Betrayal?) Dad was too much for my client. Her conversations with him whipped her up into an unbearable frenzy. She stopped seeing him in her early teens. It was not surprising that she felt that she could not keep a conversation with Dad going.

My interest in and aspirations for psychotherapy and philosophy have largely been nurtured and sustained by conversations with clients, colleagues and friends. In my account of my conversations with this young woman, I shall not neglect altogether the conversations around my work with her that helped me to make sense of my experiences.

My psychoanalytic supervisors and colleagues have often been passionate about what they refer to as 'good technique' (although If you are passionate about technique, it may not be clear just what you are in love with, other than the picture that you and people who are like you in this way do it right). These colleagues often disagree with each other about good technique and the correct interpretation. Perhaps there is more need for conversations when you are someone who not only does not know the correct interpretation or the right technique, but is also curious about making any such claims, as if to see another aspect, to make another remark is to fail at keeping the faith.

My supervisor for the client I am presenting here had his views about 'correct technique' but he did not say anything of the sort on this occasion, nor did he say something witty and knowing to the effect that my 'standing up to her' might have been driven by a fear that I might 'stand up to her'. To my confronting her as she confronted me, my mentioning her relationship with her father, he said nothing about my use of my counter-transference or my acting out. He simply said, 'Good instinct!' Then he mused about how we may be distracted by bodily beauty initially, yet once we are engaged in speaking to someone, this no longer bothers us, but we might find that someone who does not strike us initially as beautiful and desirable might become so over time. It was as if he was saying that desire is not something that is easy to predict or control, that we do not master it, and showing by his behaviour that two people can speak about desire together without one claiming to an expert on it.

The first of the six sessions with this client is not yet over, but we are now somewhere very different from where we began the session. I discovered that very soon after her father left, mother became involved with another man and pregnant. In the backward and forward of our talking to each other, she relates something that seems to be important to her and moves me before I can start to think about it. The man her mother married, her stepfather, was gentle, kind, 'very English' and a little reserved, 'nice' to her and 'sweet' to her mother. However, he was all over his own daughter, her new half-sister, as far back as my client could remember, and his daughter was all over him. It was as if they lived in a pocket of madness, noise, mess, games, jokes and laughter: giving free expression to an unquenchable appetite for each other. This was in stark contrast to the 'reserved' and controlled man my client encountered. In the evenings and weekends father and daughter were inseparable, chasing each other and play fighting -with mother shouting at them about damaging the house- playing tricks on each other and cuddled up together in front of the television, contented with each other.

As I have indicated, I heard this as a description of a full blooded passionate relationship between this daughter and father, both able to enjoy each other without too much holding back, and in contrast to my client's own relationship with her own father. As I imagined my client standing back in amazement, observing this passionate relating, I wondered aloud about her feeling left out of the wildness and mayhem. She denied this. I dropped it. Perhaps too soon to say something like this to her.

Without much in the way of prompting from me, my client spontaneously tells me (she wanted/had the desire to tell me) that once she hit her teens, she wanted to do what the other teenage girls in the area did on a Saturday night. This involved wandering around the trendy part of town wearing very little, in any weather. However, on the first Saturday night she tried to leave the house dressed as sexily as possible, her mild mannered 'English' stepfather told her in no uncertain terms that she was not leaving the house looking like that. She confronted him: 'You are not my father!' Usually a good weapon in the hands of a stepchild. He did not back down nor crumble when she opened fire. He told her firmly that she had to go and change. He was not negotiating with her. Mum, surprised at the confrontation, and catching sight of another side of her mild mannered man, tried to intervene on my client's side. He stuck to his guns. She was not leaving the house dressed like that. In the end, she had to admit defeat and change before she left the house.

This became their Saturday night ritual. She tries to argue with him. He is adamant. She tries to sneak out; he suddenly appears between her and the door. Eventually, he does not even have to say anything: he just appears and look at her; she goes upstairs and changes her clothes.

I felt that she was telling me something important to her, but I was far from clear what to make of this.

The first session is now over. I am left with a tangle of thoughts. First, that it seems that she enjoyed this more passionate and confrontational engagement with her stepfather; it was as if she had found something that was missing, that she had lost. I wondered how she experienced this. Did she feel finally held in firmly supportive arms, or was it more like enjoying hitting a brick wall? Was she saying that men who demand that she takes off her skimpy clothes now, are more exciting than men who are 'kind' and 'sweet'? Was it as if her stepfather was saying to her 'You are just too sexually exciting to be out dressed like that – I can't stand it'? Did his intervention reinforce something in apparently trying to oppose it? Second, had she temporarily stolen her stepfather's attention from her sister, and might she be heard as telling me why she does not see herself as being left out of their visceral and passionate togetherness? Might she feel that she is never left out, that she never needs to know what it is like to be without, and to be outside the walls of the city gazing inside, longing to belong, if she has the power to command attention and a response.

Middle

In her second session, dressed similarly, she explained that she had started a relationship with a 'sweet' and 'kind' young man. He sounded to me like her stepfather when he was being 'nice' rather than passionate, chasing her sister or 'standing up to' her. However, I soon found myself confused. Initially I thought this was just due to my failings, but she began to admit that she was really quite confused about it all.

Someone had told her young man that she, my client, had slept with another man. At first I thought I was being told that this was not true, a spiteful lie. Then I realised that I was being told that she had indeed slept with the man she was accused of sleeping with. I then expected to hear something about how she was overcome by her own desire and just could not resist the other man. Yet, rather than a tale of desire that erupts in spite of our efforts, a story of Eros' power, I eventually understood that she had not slept with one man but with several men, and she had not acted out of a desire for erotic pleasure with any of them.

It seemed as if she was talking about taking out insurance. She had always made it her practice not to be only with one man. She usually had a boyfriend, and at the same time she made sure that she slept with quite a few other men, not out of desire, but because when the end of her relationship came, she would know that she had always cheated: that she was not a 'mug'; that she had not been taken in by that stuff about love and romance. She would not tell the man who broke up with her what she had been up to, but she would quietly feel victorious and vindicated. I thought she wanted to convey to me that unlike the stupid people around her, she was above love and desire, whilst producing and controlling these in others.

Yet in spite of claiming to be superior and in control, she seemed to be saying that it felt different this time; but she could not say that she loved this man and it was important to her to feel loved by him. She spoke about just wanting to get him back, and wanting me, 'an expert', to help her to do this.

It was often not easy to follow her, until I began to understand that her tendency to insult and laugh at other women, and in particular the female friend of her ex-boyfriend, was designed to persuade herself that she could never lose him to a woman who is not as attractive as she is. She seemed to be contemptuous of this other woman's 'niceness'.

I said it sounded as if she thought that men were only interested in how women look, not in what they are like, or what it is like to be with them.

By the fourth and fifth sessions, there were more spaces made for reflection, for seeing how things might be related to each other, and how she may be seen as 'mistreating herself'. The latter idea seemed to interest her but she was not sure that this was so.

End

She did not show up at the beginning of her final session. I began to think that she would not come at all. Five minutes before the end of her session she appeared, apologetic. Something had happened at work and she had lost track of the time. She had rushed to at least turn up for it. She was very sorry to miss our final session. Realising that I could have given her five minutes or even fifteen, I remarked to her that this is what she does. She deprives herself and tries hard to get away from what is important. I said that I would not let her do this and miss her final session. I had a cancellation at the end of the day, and I could see her then. She left looking sad and close to tears. After she had gone, I wondered what possessed me. What was I doing? Was I behaving like the stepfather?

One of my female colleagues, who had commented each week on this client's undressed presentation asked me whether she had failed to turn up for her session.

On hearing that she was so late that I offered her the cancellation that I had, my colleague said she thought the client would not come, and that I should not have offered her another session. She had been given six sessions. She missed one. It is important that she faces the consequences of her actions. It is bad technique to offer her an extra session, to offer her something outside the contract. Who, my colleague asked, is the extra session for, the client or the therapist? So, it was technically bad and a bit 'mad'.

A conversation outside the terms of the contract

My client arrived on time for her replacement session and was soon in tears about the end of her relationship with her boyfriend. It came out that she often slipped out the back and did not do 'leaving dos'. Endings are painful and awkward, she does not know what to say or how to be. I remarked that she had tried to miss our last session; perhaps this was a way of avoiding our having to say goodbye. There were admissions of this through tears, as I tried to speak to her about how she seems to believe that she will not be liked or missed, that she has to work hard to keep men interested, and how she seems to believe her father's refrain that no man could ever love her. By always taking out insurance policies, might she contribute to her relationships failing? Perhaps, I suggested, the problem is to do with her sense of being unlovable and how she sabotages herself, how she seems to be contemptuous of her own desires to be loved.

The woman who left my consulting room seemed to be quite different to the woman who arrived for the first session. She could own feeling distressed, distraught, despairing, as well as being at war with an aspect of herself that she regarded as stupid and needy. I think of her as designing devices for dealing with love and desire, protecting herself from this kind of madness.

As always, more could be said about this client and how I worked with her. She did not want further therapy; she wanted a technique for getting her man back. I had no such thing to give her, but I could help us to get into a conversation about endings, loss and the despair she felt, her relationships with lovers and with herself. I am certainly not claiming that what I did with her is what therapists should do to all clients who turn up seriously late for a final session. I do not claim to have felt compelled to offer her another session, but to have grasped a possibility as it presented itself: the possibility of continuing our conversation about how she, in seeking to become a master of desire in others as well as herself, often proved that she was a master of self-sabotage. My official interlocutor for my work with this client, who could also speak on behalf of what is unconscious in her and in me -my supervisor- seemed not at all puzzled by my mad or inspired response to her. He could see that our conversation about how she deprives and sabotages herself might be usefully continued and taken into a different register if we had a session after she missed or forget to come to her final session.

Someone who takes a more reductive view of psychoanalysis, who feels that we have only penetrated to the heart of the matter when we are exploring the practitioner's sexual thoughts, fantasies and feelings, might be quite unsatisfied with what I have written so far. There is an important difference between a reductive psychoanalytic exploration -if not explanation- of what went on between this client and me, and on the other hand, an approach that has more to do with what Plato tries to seduce us into in *Phaedrus*. One of the ways in which my client work is connected to the conversation that is *Phaedrus* is that I am tempted to say that what has led me to philosophy and psychotherapy, and what these practices nurture in me is a passion for listening and speaking, especially -but not exclusively- when this listening and speaking is heartfelt and on the edge of what is hard to hear and engage with and hard to say or articulate. To read and to write are extensions of listening and speaking. I could have withheld my favours, following what I have been taught and siding with the part of her that wanted to stop speaking to me. I could even claim this as evidence that I am a good therapist.

Yet I was clearly not ready to end my conversation with her, or the part of her that wanted to keep speaking and listening to me, which revealed itself in her appearing at the end of her final session and at the beginning of the extra session she was given: for both of us, there was more to engage with, more to hear, more to say.

Phaedrus

'So, if the way round is long, don't be astonished: we must make this detour for the sake of things that are very important, not for what you have in mind' (Plato, 1997, p. 274)

A contemptuous attitude to loving and desiring, how they induce madness, how they rob us of our sense of being in control and reasonable, and how such feelings are inferior to a more contractual approach, is where Plato's *Phaedrus* begins. The youth Phaedrus is exceptionally handsome in a time and place where a particular social practice is well established and entrenched among some sections of the aristocracy, but by his time at least, debated, regulated and not clearly socially acceptable. In this practice, an older man -'the lover'- would receive sexual favours from a youth or young man -'the beloved'- in exchange for the young man advancing in society in some way, his receiving an education, an advantage to him and his family.

I am concerned with this complex matter here only in the context of this dialogue, where it seems that Socrates and Plato disapprove of this practice as sexual gratification but they do not disapprove of it as some sort of educational arrangement. It is certainly debatable, but they seem to disapprove of sexual acts generally, and yet, in this dialogue and the dialogue 'Symposium', they are passionately preoccupied with the erotic, with Eros, sexual love, with desiring, as if this lies at or close to the very heart of philosophy as they conceive it. Is this a contradiction or a major tension? What are we to make of this and what does it have to do with the practice of psychotherapy? Perhaps it is wise to approach such questions with caution and reverence, rather than trying to leap on them.

Meeting Phaedrus in the city, Socrates learns from him that Phaedrus' 'friend' or lover, Lysias, the best orator in Athens, has made a beautiful speech about erotic love, which is for seducing a beautiful boy, to persuade him that it is better to have sex with someone who is not in love with you than it is to have sex with someone who is in love with you.

Phaedrus and Socrates are already seduced and in love, but not with each other. Phaedrus has a powerful passion for oratory, for beautiful speeches; Socrates describes himself as 'a man who is sick with passion for hearing speeches'. (Why have I never heard one of my colleagues in the talking therapies say she has a passion for hearing people speak? Why is it that I do not say something like this? Are we bashful about our passion for listening and speaking?) They are therefore perfect for each other. Given what they are passionate about, what calls to them, they are naturally a couple, a pair. Phaedrus has found a partner for 'his frenzied dance' (Plato, 1997, 228 b).

In this dialogue and in our interactions generally, words do not always mean what they seem to mean and what people say is sometimes the opposite of what they mean or want. We play, tease, pretend, claim that we do not want what we very much want. Our partner in our dance, that involves but is not exclusively language, often catches on relatively quickly that we might not mean what we say or say what we mean. Having excited Socrates with the promise of a delicious speech, Phaedrus plays coy, pretending that he does not want to recite it. He claims not be up to the task. After all, Lysias, its author, is the best writer there is, and how could he possibly remember it all? What takes place between these two men, one young, beautiful and suited to being the beloved in an erotic relationship, the other older and suited to being the suitor or lover, should not escape the reader's attention. This dialogue begins by showing us scenes of seductive, playful, flirtatious and coy speaking, before we hear the speaking that is calculated to lead to the seduction of a physically beautiful person.

So much goes on between these two people, we might say in response to what we are shown, that it is hard to be confident that we can say what is going on. Phaedrus is tempting Socrates then being coy. Socrates tells him that he is just playing hard to get, claiming that he knows Phaedrus wants to recite the speech so much that he would force an unwilling audience to hear it. Socrates tells him to get on with it. Phaedrus protests until Socrates rightly remarks that Phaedrus is hiding a copy of the speech under his cloak. Here, perhaps, we are shown the possible discrepancy between what we claim we want and, on the other hand, what we want, and perhaps we are also being shown a connection between speaking, speeches and hiding or concealing.

They decide to leave the city, or get out from under the cloak of the city, walk along the banks of the river Llisus, to find an idyllic spot for the reading. This is the only Platonic dialogue that takes place outside the walls of the city, with only two speakers in an intimate rural setting. Might this be meaningful? As indicated above, the dialogue often seems to suggest that they could be two lovers going off to do what lovers do, but what happens is not sexual acts with bodies; two lovers of speaking and speeches speak to each other. And given that they wish to speak about desires and activities that may be outside of what the city regards as respectable, perhaps the possibility of speaking honestly and openly to each other is greatly improved by having a private conversation outside the city walls.

Can we play with this idea of being outside the walls of the city? Might we say that private conversations between people might be regarded sometimes at least as outside of the walls of the city? Do we psychotherapists think that we have private conversations outside of the walls of the city, or are our consulting rooms firmly within the city?

Two figures appear in and haunt this dialogue, and perhaps they must haunt most of our dialogues. The first is the manipulative seducer and master of technique, an expert who is firmly in control of himself as he seeks to control others, one for whom speaking is primarily about power and concealing, a figure attractive to the client I have presented. The second is one who speaks truthfully and from his soul, although in doing so he may reveal that he is a bit mad, not prudent and careful enough, dragged and driven by desires that are difficult to express or fathom. Which figure is the psychotherapist closest to? Perhaps this is a bad question. Perhaps both figures haunt our therapeutic encounters: the learned, well trained and registered practitioner, who knows how to do it by the book, and, on the other hand, one who loves to hear speaking that is truthful and from the soul, even if it is hard to make sense of this speaking.

Phaedrus begins to read the speech that is supposed to persuade someone -in this case a boy, but it need not be- that it is better to have sex with someone who is not in love with you rather than someone who is. The comic quality of these arguments often consist in the fact that they are very rational, prudent and business like. For example, someone who is in love with you might fall out of love with you, but if you are having sex with someone who is not in love with you, he cannot fall out of love with you, as he never was in love with you in the first place. Or, someone in love is mad, passion make people mad, and it is best to be wary of mad people and clearly unwise to have sex with them. And if you choose a lover from the people who are in love with you, this is likely to be a small group, but if you choose from those who are not in love with you, you are choosing from a much bigger pool. You maximise your options.

Someone who is in love with you will feel that he needs you and is hungry for you, but so what? Do you invite beggars and the hungry to your dinner party because they are the most needy? No, you grant your favours not to those who are most needy but to those who are able to give you something in return. These are arguments about economics, financial and political advantage, about why you would be stupid not to come to a 'friends with benefits' arrangement with someone who is clearly in a position to help you in return, rather than have anything to do with love and the precariousness of being loved.

Although Socrates sounds as if he is very impressed by this speech, praising it enthusiastically, it is clear to the reader and Phaedrus that Socrates is making fun of this speech and Phaedrus. We do not always say what we mean. Phaedrus is on to him and challenges him to make a better one. Now it is Socrates' turn to play hard to get and Phaedrus' turn to detect this and urge him to get on with it. Even in the face of a threat of violence from the younger, stronger man, Socrates still plays hard to get, until Phaedrus makes the worse threat he can think of, with Socrates begging him not to say it. He threatens to withhold his favours in that if Socrates does not speak, he, Phaedrus swears that he will never again recite a speech for Socrates nor ever talk to him about speeches. This lover of speeches and speaking threatens to withhold from his friend, who is sick with passion when it comes to speeches and speaking, that which seems to be central to their relationship. Complaining that he is a 'horrible man' who has said something awful but still stalling, Socrates eventually makes his speech, a better speech than Lisias', not only in that it tries to say something about what love is and what people are like, but it is more inspired and seductive, as though 'the Nymphs' madness' of the enchanted place where they are speaking to one another has taken him over, a divine madness (238d). In this speech a man who is apparently not in love with someone is persuading that person to have sex with him -Socrates introduces the possibility that this claim to not be in love might be part of the seduction, and the man might really be in love, or maybe, we might say, it could add to the seduction if this is unclear. Socrates sticks with the theme that people in love are mad and the man who is not in love is more able to be reasonable, but Socrates breaks off rather abruptly and wants to go home.

He explains, however, that he cannot leave until he has made atonement for his 'foolish and close to being impious' speech (242d), because Love is a god or something divine but defiled by foolish and dangerous speeches of the type that they have both uttered. His atonement or purification is a more involved and seductive speech, identifying that there is a divine madness 'which is a gift of the god' (244). Love is a divine madness given to us.

In this long and elaborate myth strewn speech, the soul is presented as immortal, and for humans, made up of a team of two winged horses and a charioteer. The white horse on the right is noble and well behaved, the good horse; the black horse on the left is unruly, the bad horse. Here is the tripartite structure of the soul or psyche: here is a picture of a rational mind or ego, coping with the noble and spirited white horse or superego, and on the other hand, the powerful and unruly appetites of the black horse or the id.

Much could be said here about race, psychoanalysis and the details of this elaborate speech. What needs to be said is that according to the myth, before birth the charioteer driving his winged horses is able to catch sight of what lies beyond heaven, the forms of good, beauty and justice. But because the horse on the left pulls the soul downwards, some souls fall to earth and their wings break off. Socrates argues that when the soul sees beauty, such as a beautiful body, it is reminded of the form of the beautiful that it saw beyond heaven, and it is seized with that divine madness, love, which causes the wings of the soul to begin to grow again. Bodily beauty, then, kindles or rekindles desire in us because it reminds us of something that we have glimpsed much further back than we are able to remember, back before we were born when our souls caught brief sight of the form of beauty.

I fear that it may be possible to be too literal and concrete at this point and get into an argument about whether Socrates and Plato really believe what is presented here as a myth. Maybe part of saying that something is a myth is to say that it is not a matter of literal belief. Rather than discussing Plato's metaphysics, it might be more interesting to remark that it is certainly not the same as psychoanalysis, but it might be regarded as finding an echo in psychoanalysis: namely the idea that our being in love and learning to love has much to do with our earliest relationship with our mother, being a part of her physically as well as merged with her psychologically, before our separation and sense of separateness. Loving and desiring reminds us of and echoes the life we had before our separation and individuation.

For Freud, the relationship with the father and the Oedipus complex were central to our loving and desiring. We often speak as if Klein or Winnicott or Fairbairn or Bowlby dethroned the father and helped us focus on how our loving and desiring is related to our earliest relationship with our mother. However, Otto Rank and his best friend Sandor Ferenczi, were already arguing with Freud's version of longing, loving and good technique in psychoanalysis in 1923. Rather than conceiving of the analyst as the 'stern father', they thought of the mother as being central and the analyst as being a 'midwife' helping to give birth to a new person. For Rank, the original trauma was birth and therefore the separation from mother (Breger, 2000; Coren 2001; Ferenczi, 1995).

What of my client 's relationship with her mother? Father leaves and almost immediately mother is with another man, pregnant and there is a new baby. What happened around her in her early years, and what does this have to do with the longings and desires of her parents?

Here is not the place to discuss Plato's view of the body, his idea that the superior soul is imprisoned in the tomb of the body, and what seem to be his objections to sex of any kind. But staying with our attempt to make more sense of what he might be saying, perhaps we might understand the image that love and desire water our wings as their lifting us out of foolish complacent and calculative ways of being, inspiring us to revere another person and to consider and revere our own existence. Love or being in love, then, Socrates seems to be saying, might lead us to philosophy, to speaking about what is important to us, to companionship and conversation between the people who are in love.

The client I have written about, by fighting feelings of love in herself, tried to imprison and constrain her loving and longing. They were not allowed to water her wings and encourage her to calculate less and relate more, manipulate less and appreciate more. If longing, loss, missing and mourning are part of what may break our wings, leaving us with a life focused on how we might swiftly satisfy what we experience as our needs and protect ourselves from longing and loss, Plato seems to suggest that a certain kind of conversation about loving, longing and hoping may help to restore our wings to us. When our wings are broken, we believe in and cling to the desires and fears we find ourselves with, in the way that we find ourselves with them, they help to keep us where we are and focused on their satisfaction. We are in a different place when are willing and able to move more freely in and from the place where we find ourselves, to enquiry into how we find ourselves with just these desires.

Without claiming to agree with Plato about sex, it is possible to follow the argument that Eros refers to sexual love or passionate desire, to longing and yearning, and we can insist on trying to satisfy such longings and desires as they arise, through engaging in sexual acts, but if we only dissipate and reduce Eros in this way, our lives may be poorer for it. It is as if Plato and Socrates want to say that if we follow along the line that our longing takes, if we meditate on the meaning of our desiring, wonder about our wanting, take it that talking about our desires is fundamental to beings who are often talking out loud or silently, then we have turned to philosophy, in that this practice of talking to others and ourselves, increases our capacity to reflect on what we most want or desire, and how to understand our yearnings and mourning. A problem with sex, we might say, going along with these two philosophers and in conversation with them, is that it can offer us ways of not reflecting on our cravings, not discussing our desiring, not seeing the part that our desiring and the pursuit of its satisfaction plays in our life. In this way, to reflect on and discuss Eros - longing, loving, desiring- might give our souls wings. These sorts of discussions that Plato might refer to as philosophy sometimes bear a strong resemblance to what we call psychotherapy.

The rest of this dialogue seems to be about rhetoric or oratory as the technical mastery of how to persuade, and how it is possible to confuse having some technical skill with having a profound and subtle grasp of an art. Mastering technique may be preliminary, but this is not the art itself. In the art of speaking there are many matters that do not seem to be technical and easily taught, such as that of grasping the right occasion for something, of knowing when to speak and when to hold back, the right time and timing, how to attune your hearing and speaking to the person you are speaking to(272).

One question that may arise for us is whether in the talking therapies, we give too much attention to technique, as if mastery of technique is what we need most and can be more than a preliminary, but not enough attention and thought to grasping the right occasion, timing and tact, when to speak and when to hold back, and how to attune our speaking and hearing to the individual person we are with? And perhaps what is being said here, is that these things are not so teachable.

Discussion

Many issues have been raised or touched on. Here are a few of them. The first is to do with whether we emphasise sexual acts and satisfactions when we think about the erotic, or the destructiveness of the erotic, which is arguably to follow classical psychoanalysis, or a more Kleinian version, or whether, on the other hand, the emphasis found in the Platonic dialogue we have been discussing urges us along another path. One way of speaking about this is to say that I find that I am often told that The Tango is about sex, sexual jealousy, loving and hating the same person, a battle between the man and the woman. Yet after listening to the music of this art form for well over a decade, what I heard consistently is longing and loss, laments: the lover who left me, my old sweetheart, my mother, the places I used to know that are no longer there, saying goodbye to friends and places. I have read, heard and been told many times over the last thirty years (sometimes very passionately or even aggressively), that sexual acts and fantasies, as well as aggression and destructiveness are what I need to keep my eyes and mind on when with clients. Proper technique is to do with detecting and interpreting sexual drives and fantasies, as well as our destructiveness. Yet although this is undoubtedly valuable, I often find that even when sexual feelings, acts and fantasies are prominent, I am listening to laments, to longing and loss. Sex in thoughts, fantasies and acts often seem to present itself as a way out of or substitute for what we long for. In spite of the sexual presentation of my client, I would say that longing and loss seems to be a more fruitful way to begin to think about her.

The second matter that we might want to give some thought to is whether and to what extent our conversations in the talking therapies take place outside the walls of the city. Are the talking therapies places where a person is able to speak what is in her heart and mind, although shocked and frightened by what comes out of her, a place where the usual rules, expectations and sense of what is decent and appropriate are open to conversation, if not suspended. Or on the other hand, is it the case that the walls of the city extend way beyond where the city officially ends, there is no outside of the city, and the conversation is never as open as we like to think it is?

The third possible subject for discussion is the similarities and dissimilarities between this client's attitude to Eros, to passionate desiring as something she is above and in control of, and, on the other hand, where the Phaedrus begins.

The fourth possible point of discussion is where the dialogue tries to go, namely to that tangle of Platonic notions that try to move us from trying to satisfy the desire we feel in the face of beautiful bodies to the contemplation and discussion of our passions and longing. Plato might be read as claiming that sexual activity cannot be the goal of the good life, although it may be a part of it. For Plato, keeping our eyes on the other's body cannot be as important as keeping our eyes on what he or she needs to flourish, to be well and turn out well.

Although love as a divine madness is celebrated in this dialogue, what it shows and champions is friendship, especially the friendship based around speaking, conversations, especially the speaking together that is not too intimidated by what is accepted, valued and celebrated within the walls of the city. There is the idea that we become better people through such conversations, more thoughtful, reverent and appreciative of ourselves and of others.

This paper is a reflection on two ways of being with ourselves and with others. The first way is centred around contracts, constraints, narrowly seeking to secure what we take to be our own advantage, being in control even of ourself. In this, our speaking to others is largely about how to seem, power and persuasion. It is the language of politics, policies and the city. The second way of being is a freer association with other people and ourselves (Freud, 1912), less bound by contracts, narrow conceptions of advantage, by what is thought to be the way of the city, and not without play and trickiness. This second way of being, with its passion for speaking and listening is, I have argued, crucial to one understanding of what psychotherapy is, as well as to one conception of philosophy and friendship. The friendship in Phaedrus is certainly erotic, but we miss something important about people and the desire to listen and to speak, if we insist on reducing such interactions to a desire for sexual satisfaction.

It is time to end. The heat of the sun has died down. Phaedrus suggests that they go. Socrates wants to offer up a pray to the gods of the place where their speaking has taken place. Here is his prayer.

Socrates: O dear Pan and all the other gods of this place, grant that I may be beautiful inside. Let all my external possessions be in friendly harmony with what is within. May I consider the wise man rich. As for gold, let me have as much as a moderate man could bear and carry with him.

Do we need anything else Phaedrus? I believe my prayer is enough for me.

Phaedrus: Make it a prayer for me as well. Friends have everything in common.

Socrates: Let's be off (279b-c).

Disclosure statement

No potential conflict of interest was reported by the author.

References

Breger, L. (2000). *Freud. Darkness in the midst of vision.* New York: John Wiley and Sons, Inc.

Coren, A. (2001). *Short-term psychotherapy. A psychodynamic approach.* Hampshire: Palgrave Macmillan.

Ferenczi, S. (1995). *The clinical diary of Sandor Frenczi.* Judith Dupont edited. Harvard: Harvard University Press.

Freud, S. (1912). Recommendations to physicians practising psycho-analysis. In *The standard edition of the complete psychological works of Sigmund Freud, volume XII (1911-1913): The case of Schreber, papers on technique and other works* (pp. 109–120). London: The Hogarth Press and The Institute of Psycho-Analysis

Plato. (1997). Phaedrus. In J. M. Cooper (Ed.), *Plato: complete works.* Indianapolis, IN: Hackett Publishing Company, Inc.

Is Oedipus still blind? A countertransference take on love and hate in the consulting room

Paola Valerio

ABSTRACT

This paper begins with an illustration from the HBO series 'In Treatment' and alludes to the gender bias in the portrayal of male and female analysts' erotic counter-transference on screen. The author includes several clinical vignettes from her clinical practice, taking a critical stance on the use of the oedipal myth as a concept or tool in analytic treatment. It is suggested that we need to turn this myth on its head in the consulting room as well as on screen, and see that the analyst may be the one who is blind; who needs to own up to her own desires in treatment.

Every new arrival on this planet is faced with the task of mastering the Oedipus complex; anyone who fails to do so falls a victim to neurosis. With the progress of psycho-analytic studies the importance of the Oedipus complex has become more and more clearly evident; its recognition has become the shibboleth that distinguishes the adherents of psychoanalysis from its opponents.

Sigmund Freud, footnote added to 1914 edition of *Three Essays on Sexuality* (1905).

In the popular American HBO series, 'In Treatment', the actor Gabriel Byrne plays Dr Paul Weston, an unhappily married psychoanalyst in his fifties. Interestingly, whilst female analysts are often portrayed as love -starved individuals who need to be rescued by their male patients, no comparable caricature of male therapists is apparent in the male dominated film industry, which often depicts the male analyst, rather like Paul, as a victim of his sexually dangerous disturbed female patients.(Lane, 1995; Valerio, 2004)

I have found the In Treatment series useful as a teaching tool. It is dated, but seems to have remained popular and is therefore well known to students. The main protagonist, Paul, is portrayed as a struggling 'wounded healer' sort, although in this case, as generally competent. The protagonist's struggles in maintaining boundaries with his 'seductive' and/or inquisitive clients, may well resonate with many therapists, which will be explored further in clinical illustrations below.

This paper is developed from a presentation about love and desire in the consulting room which was given at a recent conference on Love, Sex and Psychotherapy in a Post Romantic Era. I began by asking participants to watch two short clips from In Treatment, an exercise I often use when teaching about the erotic countertransference. Students are asked to observe a few minutes from two different episodes or sessions, with two different patients; Mia and Laura. In each episode both women confess their love and desire for their analyst, Paul.

Firstly, Laura a year into treatment, the scene begins: She arrives for her session, beautiful, dishevelled, dressed simply, tastefully and very sexily in black, smudged make-up, ripped tights. She confesses her longing, her desire for her therapist, 'How long have you felt this way' Paul asks, almost accusingly.

{Interestingly, there is also a teaching version of this Laura clip on YouTube, in which an American male, possibly a psychoanalyst, with a rather disembodied voice, comments in a rather surreal manner with moral overtones (as if Paul really is a therapist and Laura a real patient) on Paul's lack of technical skills in the face of Laura's 'cheap trips'; for example, 'deliberately ripping her pantyhose, smudged mascara, pretending to be sick etc in order to seduce Paul'.}

'That's not the answer I was looking for' ... Laura continues; 'what was the reply you were looking for?' Paul asks? Laura continues to tell Paul about her longings in two graphic scenarios. He almost collapses listening to the version which ends with making love and it is clear from her voice and posture this is rich sex. Paul can hardly contain himself, he shifts uneasily in his chair, struggling to return her gaze. He exudes desire and his bodily language and tone of voice cannot disguise this. ... 'I'm not an option' he says, ... the parameters and ethics are clearly defined ... 'I'm your therapist'.

Second clip, another session, another scene. This time Mia arrives, now pregnant, plump, more casually dressed, possibly no longer an object of desire, or so she laments. She jokes with Paul, 'now I am fat' she asks ... can I still get the drooling guy in the back of the six o'clock train?"

And so, it continues 'Can we call it a day and go to a bar and get drunk?' Mia asks. Paul flirts back, playfully, 'is that the bar in Soho where you hoped we'd run into each other?' ...... and so forth for a while amicably.

'But seriously' she asks, after a while, now moving beyond the symbolic to the real, indeed to her very real fear of raising a child by herself and her acute loneliness. 'Will you help me .... will you be a father to my child'. 'A father?' Paul replies rather concretely.

'You know what I mean' she replies ... 'Will you help me? I'm scared. I've never done this before .... you're a father, you have children.'

I ask participants two questions. Firstly, what is the difference between these interactions or the two different scenarios, since both patients attempt to 'seduce' the therapist? Secondly, what might Paul have said to Laura instead of the formulaic – 'I'm your therapist ... I am not an option?'

Without fail the responses to question one are similar, across trainings and practitioners (for example integrative counsellors, psychologists and analytic psychotherapists). Students generally note that the main difference between the sessions is in the atmosphere in the consulting room, despite the similarity in advances to the therapist. In the session with Laura it is tense, uncomfortable, even pathologizing, they note. Yet they also try to dissect Laura's history to explain her attempts to seduce Paul and hence why this session is so uncomfortable. Whereas they note that the session with Mia, in contrast, is comfortable, relaxed, playful even flirtatious.

Responses to the second questions usually vary from stating that Paul was correct to state the boundaries to Laura, to suggestions that perhaps he could have alluded to her father issues, such as Paul being a father substitute. Some students who have seen the series, allude to Laura's childhood sexual abuse. Paul should refer to her need to trade sex in return for love or intimacy, they add. (1)

In response I may comment that none of these interpretations are incorrect and may need to be said at some point in a timely and therapeutic manner. But how might this capture what is happening in the session rather than pathologise Laura and deny what had been created between them, for whatever reason? Is there ever any advantage or therapeutic gain to a sharing of the real, especially when it is so obvious? Or would this be abusive or conversely a 'triumph' for the patient?

Could Paul have said to Laura something like, "Gosh if a young woman like you approached me outside of therapy I would be immensely flattered, but we both know this is forbidden between us. Yet, the fact that it is happening here in therapy makes me wonder about how we can understand this together. It reminds me of what you have previously told me about some of the dangerous but exciting relationships with men you have been drawn into but how this has always ended up with you feeling abused".

(1) In this paper I am preoccupied with underrepresentation in the literature of accounts of the analyst's unresolved longings and lust and a gender bias in a key construct in psychoanalytic formulation, the Oedipus complex. There is not space to discuss fully the severe impact on clients of sexual abuse or professional boundary violations, Nor does this paper address the ineffectiveness or inappropriateness of traditional psychoanalytic psychotherapy in work with survivors of abuse where there are serious issues in relation to trust, memory construction and disorganised attachments. I have written about this elsewhere (Valerio, 2011; Valerio & Lepper, 2009, 2010)

Such a response might have invited an adult to adult interaction in which Paul could safely acknowledge his attraction to Laura, which in the light of her stunning presence, might be hard to avoid. Yet, how does one achieve this safely and therapeutically? Of course, in the second scenario there is a more playful dynamic, an 'as if' quality to the material in which the erotic becomes transformative because Paul is not struggling with his erotic countertransference. With Mia he is not troubled by denial of his lust and longings.

We are familiar with Freud views on the transference:

'If the patient's advances were returned it would be a great triumph for her, but a complete defeat for the treatment. She would have succeeded in what all patients strive for in analysis – she would have succeeded in acting out, in repeating in real life, what she ought only to have remembered, to have reproduced as psychical material and to have kept within the sphere of psychical events ... ... The love relationship in fact destroys the patient's susceptibility to influence from analytic treatment. A combination of the two would be an impossibility ... ' (Freud, 1915)

Freud was influenced in his formulation of transference by significant events with his colleague and friend Dr Joseph Breuer and Breuer's patient Anna O. These encounters contributed to his retreat from the hypothesis of seduction and incest towards a hypothesis of the child as seducer, which was operationalised in the Oedipus myth. We may be less aware that his thinking about countertransference was influenced by his encounter with Jung, in the intense period of friendship between the two men, and following Jung's affair with Sabine Spielrein, as documented in the Freud-Jung letters.

Freud advised Jung to 'dominate his countertransference' (McGuire, 1974). The countertransference was something to be mastered; the analyst must remain anonymous so as not to contaminate the transference and allow the patient to seduce him.

To what extent are we influenced by the Oedipus myth and seduction theory today? It seems incredibly difficult to shake off and to reappraise its relevance. And if so how much does this enduring myth castrate the therapist and humiliate our patients? Are psychoanalysts still trained to believe our patients will fall in love with us and is far less attention paid to any reciprocal feelings or any unresolved needs we might have to be loved? Searles (1959) rather radically for his time questioned this fear and anxiety around the erotic countertransference, even among seasoned analysts, openly admitting that he falls in love with each one of his patients:

"Since I began doing psycho-analysis, I have found, time after time, that during the work with every one of my patients who has progressed to, or very far toward, a thoroughgoing analytic cure, I have experienced romantic and erotic desires to marry, and fantasies of being married to, the patient'. (p. 180)

Yet the idea that we develop erotic and sexual longings for our patients and do so very commonly indeed, is still not acknowledged openly in most clinical trainings and I believe it is not just a problematic area in psycho-analytic trainings.

Soon after qualifying, admittedly some time ago now, I began seeing a patient several times a week, an attractive lesbian woman in her forties. She told me that she had fallen in love with me and was very open in her attempts to win me over, mostly in a charming manner. As she was very artistic she would bring me poems and songs she had written and paintings. I did the usual job of interpreting her love and need to be special with me as a replacement for the loving mother/therapist that she had never had as a child. I wondered with her about her devotion and care of her ailing mother, and we discussed how hurtful it was that her mother always preferred her neglectful younger sister. She had no contact with her father. Her relationship history to date was of getting involved with abusive women. Several years into intensive therapy, she met her future long-term partner, a beautiful, intelligent heiress in her thirties. Yet, although I was delighted for my patient for sure, and felt somewhat smugly that the therapy had been successful, I was suddenly aware of an unexpected sense of loss, something I had not expected. Slowly it crept upon me; a realisation that I had also taken great pleasure in her attention, now the province of another. I felt replaced! Yet I could not recall being trained to expect that I might be the victim in this newly created oedipal triangle. I had been led to expect only that I might have to resist the patient, certainly not that I might experience a desire for such seduction? Was my response unusual or worse unprofessional, or is this a rather common occurrence?

How we experience, perceive and speak of love in treatment is culturally relevant (Foucault, 1976) My ideas about the nature of love also influenced my idea of a 'successful ending' with my patient who entered a loving monogamous alliance. In the psychoanalytic literature we are perhaps more able nowadays to acknowledge the erotic countertransference, but we are still far more tolerant and tolerated, when owning up to erotic feelings that are loving, and less likely to acknowledge the hateful version of the erotic. Simon (2018) presented a paper at this conference, highlighting research which suggests that therapists may become even more anxious about erotic feelings when working with adolescents. A taboo area no doubt enforced by safeguarding issues. Yet adolescents repeatedly push at the boundaries invoking love, lust, anger and hatred in equal measure.

In his seminal paper Winnicott (1949) observed the therapeutic value of hate and as practitioners we must also work with hateful attempts at seduction. I first became aware of my limited understanding in working with more hateful versions of the erotic countertransference with my first training patient, Lucy, a woman who looked somewhat eerily like the series character Laura. Lucy stirred up a huge amount of lustful and sexual material early on in treatment and I soon realised that I was at sea.

Any suggestion of hatred and sexual excitement with our patients creates extreme guilt in all practitioners, since acting out this excitement is against our code of ethics. More so if we feel that what might excite us is also 'perverse.' Things have improved for sure, but therapists who admit to any desire with clients are often seen at best as unprofessional and at worst predatory. Such an illicit sense of shame silences us and our trainees, mirroring the secrets world experienced by many of our analysands who are survivors of sexual abuse; whose bodies may have responded with arousal to the violation from perpetrators, creating a deep cavate of buried shame (Diamond & Valerio, 2018)

As a newly qualified analyst, I was surprised by my initial response to Lucy early 'in treatment'. With Lucy, whose full history is documented elsewhere (Valerio, 1997) my attempts to defend against my hateful feelings resulted in a type of 'proper' but I came to realise 'pseudo' therapy in which I was not owning my own part. In 1997, Joy Shaevarien wrote an illuminating paper, followed by an edited book (Schaverien, 1997, 2006), which explores erotic enactments in same sex dyads. In her paper she suggests that the cultural lens is predominately focused on the male therapist/female dyad. Shaevarien argues that women therapists are far more comfortable talking about pre-oedipal dynamics with men, than in acknowledging the real adult to adult erotic tensions in the room, resulting in a pattern she observed of 'men who leave to soon'. This idea was relevant in my work with Lucy. Time and time again I have found in working with trainees how in sanitising rather than dealing with the real erotic tensions with their patients, men (and women) complain that they feel infantilised or patronised, even pathologised and hence become ashamed of their longings. This will often end the therapy prematurely.

My patient Lucy arrives for her session, still struggling with depression and drug abuse. The following extract is after 15 months of intensive Jungian analysis:

She arrives, late, eyes swollen and mascara-stained, long hair tousled and exuding the heavy odour of stale tobacco. She looks delicate, almost beautiful, but like a photograph, a still image in time. She is dressed, as often, in muddy and murky clothes, dull bluey-grey, the colour of a dead child's eyes. I feel that the space between us is pregnant with a stillborn child, She begins the session by telling me that she feels as if she is in a dream. 'I know that you said things might feel worse when I started to give up the medication' . . . . . . she speaks softly.

Her voice begins to shake and she bursts into tears, throbs, but I notice her control, her breathing, her body remains rigid, constricted. She continues 'I know you will think I'm pathetic. I feel pathetic I feel disgusted with myself, it's all about sex just as it was with William' . She began to describe the sexual encounter to me, but her account was of a partial nature -part disclosures, part fragments of traumatic memories, which left me feeling eventually frustrated and tantalized, angry perhaps, strangely excluded but perhaps also aroused.

In response to her tears, my earlier images of being with a corpse, feelings of hopelessness, evaporate. I feel an immense rage surge within. I realize I want to murder my patient. The idea shocks me. My violent image shames me. I am, of course, aware of the implied criticism, it is my fault that she feels this way but this does not seem to fully explain my response. I realise that I feel penetrated by her and somewhat uncomfortably, excited at the same time.

Stoller (1975) has written about 'perversion', a term I use cautiously, as the "erotic form of hatred', about making hate rather than love; of the encounter in which the patient reverses the abusive experience, attempting to seize power by turning the tables on the therapist who inexplicably now feels excited and abused. Khan (1979), Glasser (1986) and Weldon (1988) among others have contributed to our understanding of these dynamics in the clinical encounter and yet we hear so many accounts of 'perverse' patients, without the sub plot -the therapist's perversions or struggles. (Valerio, 2002, 2004) .

Another analysand, Sally, a 42-year-old barrister who was referred to me for further work, described a history of sexual and emotional abuse with male partners as a young woman and childhood neglect from her depressed mother and absent father. After only a week of seeing me, she had to postpone starting weekly therapy due to her daughter's illness. The following week when she arrived for her session, a truly bizarre turn of events occurred (which I am reticent and ashamed to admit publicly). She arrived on time but somehow, I had forgotten about her, but most worryingly I completely failed to recognize her, and then to top it all finally mistook her for my new cleaner, (whom to be fair I was expecting but I had not yet met). Instead of leading Sally to my consulting room, I promptly showed her into my private space whilst alluding to the ironing, adding "you look familiar! Surprisingly once I/we suddenly reconnected in role, I realizing just why she looked familiar, she bravely accepted my invitation to remain for the session, and we somehow began a process of digesting this embarrassing incident, a process which has continued in following sessions. She was able to discuss how it felt, to be both forgotten about and treated in such a bizarre way. An intelligent, psychologically minded woman, she reflected that it was as if she had stepped back in time and that she was with her 'mad mother' again, but most significantly, she also felt responsible 'to make it right' rather than allow herself to be furious with me, instead she was able to see psychologically, eyes 'wideshut', she later said to me 'only noticing red and purple cushions' "in the front room, she added, 'no photos or pictures' or anything personal. A further enactment of her childhood relationship with her mother, whom she had protected.

Somewhat later I managed to reflect on the way I had also put myself in a vulnerable position. I began to understand that somehow, I had enacted her oedipal dynamic allowing her entry to the forbidden parental space, a chamber of usually very tightly closed doors. She had spoken of many long car journeys when her father took her back to her childhood home in

France. Together as a couple they would talk about serious and intimate matters that were outside of the comprehension of her mother, who was both depressed and less academic. This always made her feel uncomfortable, collusive. I understood later that there must have been a complimentary dynamic on some level with this engaging woman which had facilitated this enactment. I had to reflect on my own part and why I had also ultimately ended up as an intrusive, abusive analyst, breaking boundaries with my analysand. This seemed important, we had focused on why she has been told by her partner that she makes men, feel powerless and often causes them to act 'out of character'. She confided that they complain about being pushed into behaving in disturbing ways, driven mad with jealously, but that she has no real idea about what she might do to provoke them. Interestingly she advised me that she never has this dynamic with women, although clearly as a woman I had also been drawn in.

Contemporary debates in psychoanalytic thinking focus on the advantages and disadvantages of adopting a more open stance with patients. Although one criticism of this approach which is associated with the relational school, as discussed in Loewenthal (2014) is that there may now be too much of a focus on the analyst, therein feeding our narcissism which is not in service of the patient.

As a result of developments in neuroscience, clinicians are now more aware of the inevitably of enactments with patients and the idea that psychotherapy is less of a 'talking cure' and more of a relational interaction. (Stern, 2005). We understand that where there has been early trauma, bodily memory or implicit relational knowing is primarily accessed in the consulting room and often this manifests in very difficult or heated encounters, wherein boundaries between therapist and analysand may indeed become 'sloppy'. In such situations we are indeed drawn in to role playing elements of the clients and our own history (Diamond & Valerio, 2018)

This encounter with my patient also caused me to reflect on Jung's ideas about gender in this oedipal drama. Jung (1946) was the first to suggest as a supplement to the Oedipus complex, the Electra Complex, emphasizing not just the phallic organization and cathexis of the libido but the little girl's previous attachment to the mother. Freud saw us as moving in a linear fashion towards specific genders in sexual development, and at the same time recognising the polymorphous potential in physical desire, Jung saw development of libido as part of a bigger picture where we discover both our feminine and masculine selves, an interplay and identification with both mother and father, anima and animus, and thereby finding a way towards something nearing wholeness or completeness.

In relation to my patient I eventually came to feel that I had been drawn into an enactment of the father's part; perhaps not so only as the mad mother but also as the powerful intrusive father. Perhaps this anima/

animus idea may help us to be more gender fluid around oedipal dynamics, at least if we can allow ourselves to receive and constellate both anima and animus projections. The difficulty is that our fear of difference is as equally powerful as our need to realise ourselves, since any relationship be it heterosexual, homosexual, bisexual, transsexual, or other binary combination, so often proves to be a battle of opposites for men and women.

In the Oedipus myth the emphasis is on the crime of the banished one, Oedipus, but there is much less of a focus on parental neglect, on the sins of fathers and mothers; on lust and abuse in sending him away in the first place. Moreover, in the Sophocles' version, it is suggested that Jocasta knew of her son's identity and woefully commits incest.

In a similar fashion, I would argue that therapists need to become aware of how they interpret their patients' erotic and aggressive wishes, often without considering their own participation. The analysand's transference cannot be separated from the analyst's countertransference, both are mutually constructed, and hence the very notion of 'counter' is questionable (Gaitanidis, 2018). In looking at love in the consulting room, as well as on screen, both in its erotic and 'so called perverse' manifestations, I would conclude with the question of whose blindness really needs to be addressed?
Perhaps, as Kristeva suggests;

> The analyst occupies that place of the Other;
>
> he is a subject that is supposed to know.
>
> and know how to love and as a consequence he will, in the cure,
>
> become the supreme loved one and the first-class victim

(Kristeva, 1987, p. 13)

Disclosure statement

No potential conflict of interest was reported by the author.

References

Diamond, N. & Valerio, P. (2018). Between bodies – Working in the liminal zone. In P. Valerio (Ed.), *Introduction to countertransference in therapeutic practice; A myriad of mirrors* (Chapter 1, p. 38). Routledge.

Foucault, M. (1976). *The history of sexuality. Vol 1 The will to knowledge.* Edition Galimard.

Freud, S. (1915). Observation on transference love (Further Recommendations on the Technique of Psycho-analysis III,)

Gaitanidis, A. (2018). The so-called 'counter-transference' and the mystery of the therapeutic encounter'. In P. Valerio (Ed.), *Introduction to countertransference in therapeutic practice; A myriad of mirrors* (Chapter 13, pp. 221–229). Routledge.

Glasser, M. (1986). Identifications and its vicissitudes as observed in the perversions. *International Journal of Psycho-Analysis, 67,* 9–16.

Jung, C. G. (1946). The psychology of the transference. In *Collected works* (Vol. 16). London: Routledge & Kegan Paul.

Khan, M. (1979). *Alienations in perversions.* London: Karnac.

Kristeva, J. (1987). *Tales of love.* New York, NY: Columbia University Press.

Lane, R. C. (1995). Incomplete mourning. Betrayal, and revenge in the price of tides: Erotic countertransference in the cinema. *Journal of Contemporary Psychotherapy, 25*(2), 123–134.

Loewenthal, D. (Ed.). (2014). *Relational psychotherapy, psychoanalysis and counselling: Appraisals and reappraisals.* Routledge.

McGuire, W. (Ed.). (1974). *The Freud/Jung letters: The correspondence between Sigmund Freud and Carl Jung.* Princeton, NJ: Princeton University Press.

Schaverien, J. (1997). Men who leave too soon. *British Journal of Psychotherapy, 14*(1), 3–16.

Schaverien, J. (Ed.). (2006). *Gender, countertransference and the erotic transference.* Routledge.

Searles, H. F. (1959). Oedipal love in the counter transference. *International Journal of Psycho-Analysis, 40,* 180–190.

Simon, L. (2018) *What makes it difficult for psychodynamic psychotherapists to work with adolescent sexuality-a thematic exploration.* Conference Presentation. Love Sex and Psychotherapy in a Post romantic Era. Roehampton University

Stern. (2005). The 'something more' than interpretation revisited: Sloppiness and co-creativity in the psychoanalytic encounter. *Journal of the American Psychoanalytic Association, 53*(3), 693–729.

Stoller, R. J. (1975). *Perversion; the erotic form of hatred.* London: Karnac.

Valerio, P. (1997). Secret friends: Borderline symptomatology and post-traumatic stress disorder in a case of reported sexual abuse. *British Journal of Psychotherapy, 14*(1), 18–32.

Valerio, P. (2002). Love and hate: A fusion of opposites: A window to the soul. In D. Mann (Ed.), *Love and hate psychoanalytic perspectives 2004* (Chapter 15, pp. 253–267). Routledge.

Valerio, P. (2004). Broken boundaries: Perverting the therapeutic frame. Ch. 7. In M. Luca (Ed.), *The therapeutic frame* (pp. 116–127). London: Taylor Francis.

Valerio, P. (2011). Who let the boys in? Discussion of a mixed gender group for victims of sexual abuse. *British Journal of Psychotherapy, 27*(1), 79–92.

Valerio, P., & Lepper. (2010). Change and process in long and short term groups for survivors of child abuse. *Group Analysis, 43*(1), 31–49.

Valerio, P., & Lepper, G. (2009). Taylor & Francis. Sorrow shame and self-esteem perception of self and others in groups for survivors of child sexual abuse. *Psychoanalytic Psychotherapy*, *23*(2), 136–153.

Weldon, E. (1988). *Mother, Madonna, Whore: The idealization and denigration of motherhood*. London: Karnac.

Winnicott, D. (1949). Hate in the counter-transference. *International Journal of Psycho-Analysis*, *30*, 69–74(IJP).

(No) time for love: Reflecting on relationships in psychotherapy

Poul Rohleder

ABSTRACT

This paper presents a response to the six papers comprising this special issue on Love, Sex and Psychotherapy in a Postromantic Era. The theme of temporality is explored in reading the papers: specifically, time in terms of self-other development and the capacity to relate to others as a separate subjectivity, the social and cultural context in which we are situated, and temporality in psychotherapy. In responding to the papers, it is argued that psychoanalysis perhaps never was a 'romantic' endeavour, recognising as it does the fantasies and fictions involved in the idea of unconditional, and everlasting love. Rather, it recognises the role of being able to tolerate love and hatred in the experience of intimate relationships, whatever its forms.

In reading the six papers that have been included in this special issue, temporality seems to me an important aspect to reflect on when thinking about relationships. It is implicated in various ways in all the papers, and in my response I would like to bring together my reading of the different papers by reflecting on different notions of temporality that I think have been touched on. That is: time in terms of self-other development and the capacity to relate to others as a separate subjectivity; the social and cultural context in which we are situated; and temporality in psychotherapy .

When I was asked to be a respondent, time was also of the essence. I had a relatively short period of time to read the papers, reflect on them and write my response. I did not want to rush, but there was a need to act and put down words. It has made me think that our experience and understanding of relationships has a lot to do with our experience and tolerance of time.

Relationships are defined by time. We celebrate anniversaries that define relationships – when they began and when they ended. We equate relationships with love, and their beginnings and endings are marked by the notion of love – when we fall in love, and when we fall out of love. The time in-between is where the real 'work' of relationships is. This might be what Freud referred to as 'common unhappiness'. Love, as the papers rightly suggest, involve fantasies and fiction. The word romance comes from its French root, *romanz*, referring to a narrative or story. In thinking about relationship, there is, perhaps, a need to separate 'fact' from fiction. A question that may be reflected by the so-called post-romantic era is: Do we have time for love?

Developing the capacity to relate to others as a separate subjectivity

All of the papers, to a greater or lesser degree, emphasise the need to take time to understand relationship(s) and their meanings. The papers draw on various psychoanalytic theories, to observe that our capacity to have relationships with others involves the development of subjectivity and the capacity to relate to others as separate objects with their own minds.... At risk of repeating some of the theories that the papers have already referred to, I draw on psychoanalytic theories within the British object relations school which emphasise the development of the capacity for relationships and 'mature' love as linked to the developmental psychic separation of the infant from their mother. Winnicott (1960) famously stated that 'there is no such thing as an infant' (p.586); there is only an infant and maternal care (mother) as a merged state of oneness. The mother spends time with the infant in a state of reverie (Bion, 1962), where the mother absorbs the infant's mental state into her own mind and transforms the projection into something that the infant can use and assimilate. Through this process of containment, the infant is able to develop a capacity to tolerate frustration and separation. As the infant matures, the child moves from relating to their mother as a narcissistic extension of themselves, where all their desire and aggression is projected into, to experiencing and perceiving the mother as a separate object. In this stage, the object is not the all loving good object that provides all that is needed, nor is it the evacuated hated bad object; it is both. Klein (1946) formulated this as the depressive position, where the child can tolerate its ambivalent feelings towards the object; as the object of love who nurtures, as well as being the object of hate who frustrates.

Helen Gilbert's 'Should Love be Unconditional' reminds us that some family relationships and parent-child relationships are not loving. We know that the notion of 'unconditional love' of parent and family is often a fiction, as in some family relationships hate (more than love) resides. This can be observed in the experiences of abuse, cruelty, even murder within families. It is the children of parents who may have not been 'good-enough' parents (Winnicott, 1965) who we are most likely to see in our consulting rooms.

Winnicott, expanding on the inter-relational aspect of the mother-child relationship, argued how a child can only properly be in a relationship with the mother as a separate being, and be able to 'use' her, after the infant destroys the merged mother and experiences her as a relatable object: 'The object, if it is to be used, must ... be real in the sense of being part of a shared reality, not a bundle of projections.' (Winnicott, 1969, p. 712). This period of separation from a merged state is fundamental for our capacity to know ourselves as individuals, and to relate to others as persons in their own right. As Birksted-Breen (2016) states: 'the time of separation which brings distress is *also* the time which can promote psychic development' (pg. 145). Most of the papers refer to desire being linked to the longing to return back to the merged infant-mother state, where all our narcissistic needs are met. However, this desire may be riddled with all sorts of fictions and fantasies about relationships and love. The papers make some reference to the development of subjectivity to observe the difference between 'mature' object relating and narcissistic object relating. While the separation of self from object is a developmental achievement, there is a recognition that we may oscillate between merged and more separate states of relating. Some merger with the object may be adaptively necessary in forming a new relationship, but for mutuality and 'love' to exist, each party also needs to be able to oscillate away from merged states to be able to relate to each other as separate subjectivities. To be in a relationship with someone involves time and the continuity and survival of the object (Birksted-Breen, 2016). Anthony McSherry in 'A phenomenology of love, thanks to Lacan, Miller, and Jellybean' quotes Miller, who claims that "we love the one who seems to harbour the answer to our question, 'Who am I?'" This takes a phenomenological exploration of the subject's experience with the object. This formulation of love draws on Lacan's notion of the mirror, which Winnicott (1971) in turn develops to refer to the (m)other as a mirroring object. The infant learns who they are, as reflected in the eyes, face and affective responses of the (m)other. However, when the infant moves from a narcissistic object relating to recognise the (m)other as a separate subject, they come to ask: 'Who are you?'. It is at this time that anxiety, insecurity and unhappiness may prevail; as reflected by McSherry in his paper when referring to the anxiety of one trying to figure out 'what the other wants from me' (special issue page number).

Bollas (2013) argues that the capacity for perceptive identification (the awareness of the integrity of the object) – as opposed to projective identi-fication where the object is a narcissistic extension of the self – is a necessary capacity for 'mature' love, as it allows for 'a true depth of intimacy with the object, which is loved for its own sake and not because it reflects the self' (Nettleton, 2017, p. 49). Relationships involve working through desire, as well as hate, aggression, and guilt (as in Klein's depres-sive position), and responding to the desire of the other. And as Paola

Valerio in 'Is Oedipus still Blind?' reminds us, some erotic relationships may involve hate. Anthony McSherry in 'A phenomenology of love, thanks to Lacan, Miller, and Jellybean' suggests that relationships involve repair work: 'it is the endless questioning and uncertainty that seems to be important, seems to indicate an ontological uncertainty at the heart of the experience of love' (special issue page number). Similarly, Onel Brooks in 'Conversations outside the walls of the city: techniques, erotic love and the wings of desire in Phaedrus and psychotherapy' argues that love involves moving from a longing and desire for merger to separateness, involving 'companionship and conversation' about our wanting and desires, as well as our disappointments and losses with the person(s) we love.

What about polyamory?

In its focus on the relationship, does psychoanalysis have 'romantic' notions of relationships as privileging monogamy. No doubt it does. Does monogamy belong to the 'romantic' era and polygamy to the 'post-romantic'? In framing the question in this way, it suggests monogamy as a fiction, a fantasy. It seems to me that we should not easily moralise one being 'better' and 'healthier' than the other. It is not the nature of the relationship that needs to be 'diagnosed', it is the quality of relating, and what relationships mean for the client. This seems to be the position of the authors of these papers.

'Polyamory- a romantic solution to Wanderlust?' is the only paper that really considers polyamory. The paper seems to have some sympathy for polyamory. It points out that polyamory, rooted in open dialogue about relational contracts, may provide an honesty in a relationship. It also points out how the very acts of contracting and timetabling (features of polyamorous relationships) may be the very things that bring estranged monogamous couples back together – making time for each other, for sex, for conversation. Time to be together. However, one might also ask if in certain polyamorous relationships, the nature of timetabling is different: timetabling time to spend apart (and with someone else).

This brought to my mind a client, who seemed to spend a lot of time with the primary partner discussing and arguing over timetabling multiple relationships, and how to define each of them. There were conflicts over whether a secondary relationship was more intimate than it should contractually be or not; too much time spent with one and not the other. As we explored in therapy, there seemed to be less time for the primary partners to discuss other things, including what may actually be going on in their relationship. Of the clients of mine who have been in open or polyamorous relationships, it was apparent that these were renegotiated relationships, once sex and intimacy stopped. Thus, it is important to consider what is, and what is not, being worked through in the relationship? Anthony McSherry asks whether marriage attempts to put an end to the uncertainty of love and relationships by contracting into a fictional 'happily ever after'. Could we sometimes say the same for polyamory, where uncertainty about 'who I am to you' gets diluted into the fictional security and acceptance of having to only be 'part of me to part of you'?

We cannot generalise from the consulting room to all relationships. We know the dangers of this in the way that homophobic psychoanalysts formulated homosexuality on the basis of their distressed gay patients (Lewes, 2009): Homosexuality is a pathology; my homosexual patient has a pathology; thus, homosexuality is a pathology. I reflect here on my clients experiencing problems in their relationships, who happen to be in open relationships or polyamorous relationships.

Our social and cultural context

The call for papers for this special issue raises questions about the consideration of time: do we as psychotherapist hold values about 'healthy' relationships that belong to this era, or a past era? Are we romantic, or can we be, should we be, post-romantic? What is this era that we find ourselves in? The papers, while questioning whether some psychoanalytic theories (e.g. the Oedipus complex) are no longer relevant, did not seem to really consider the social and cultural era that we find ourselves in.

All the papers are located in 'western' contemporary thought. Helen Gilbert's 'Should Love be Unconditional' and Marian O'Connor's 'Polyamory- a romantic solution to Wanderlust?' explicitly refer to contemporary 'western' culture, that is defined by increased individualism (Gilbert), and social and economic uncertainty (O'Connor). Many psychosocial theorists have described contemporary 'western' culture as a culture of narcissism, linked to capitalism and neoliberalism (e.g. Layton, 2011). They describe a society marked by the decline of the family and social structure, and the promotion of the individual as consumer and agent of their own wellbeing. In this contemporary culture we value individualism and autonomy, of the sort that devalues emotionality and interdependence, and instead inadvertently promotes 'radical aloneness' (Layton, 2011, p. 114).

Alongside this, we are living in a contemporary era of immediacy. We have instant news; instant online lives. Lemma (2017) reflects on what impact this culture of immediacy may have on relationships. She writes about the 'disintermediation' of relating; cutting out the 'middle-man' (time?) and getting immediate gratification, which she argues resonates with the merged infant-mother relationship of early life. She considers the importance of some delay of the gratification of desire for the development of subjectivity. Lemma states, 'desire is measured in terms of time: it is about anticipation and the delay of gratification' (pg. 66). Lemma distinguishes between what she refers to as an often 2D(esire) contemporary world of instantaneous gratification: Desire leading to instant Delivery of gratification, in contrast to a 3D(esire) world where Desire is followed by Delay, and eventual Delivery of gratification. This space and time of delay, which we might consider akin to the important space for reverie and for reflection, is important for the development of subject-object relating. Does this culture of immediacy risk some relationships becoming more 2-dimensional?

Relationships, in some ways, have also become objects for consumption – swipe right for yes, left for no. Some of my clients who make use of online dating Apps talk with frustration, and despair, of 'not feeling it' on the first, maybe second date, and not being able to find a partner. If 'the spark' is not there, then there is a swift moving on. Some of this is the chase of the fantasy and fairy tale of 'love'. However, they talk of an increased urgency for the 'spark' to be there straight away; there is no time for it to develop. Increasingly, such Apps are not only being used to meet a potential partner, but rather to hook up to have sex. Open relationships in many ways are made more possible by them. It is not my intention here to make this a moral issue. There is nothing necessarily wrong with casual, anonymous sex. However, in thinking about love and relationships, it is not uncommon for some to confuse sex for love. Onel Brooks in 'Conversations outside the walls of the city: techniques, erotic love and the wings of desire in Phaedrus and psychotherapy' drawing on the philosophies of Plato and Socrates, suggests that sex may 'offer us ways of not reflecting on our cravings, not discussing our desiring, not seeing the part that our desiring and the pursuit of its satisfaction plays over time' (special issue page number).

Sally Parsloe in 'Romance and Murder' concludes by asking whether in the post-romantic era we use relationships (others) in a delusional, collusive way to perpetuate the fictions we have about ourselves. One might bask in the love of the number of followers or 'friends' one has on social media, how many likes, and how many expressions of interest to hook up. It may give us the illusion of popularity and being desired. Nevertheless, it may keep us alienated. It may be no wonder that loneliness is on the rise (Gil, 2014).

Polyamory has always existed, but there is a new cultural interest in polyamory, fluidity and openness. It is a shift towards breaking down the tyranny of norms. Queer theory disrupts the notion of 'identity'; arguing for a state of fluidity rather than fixity; and challenging the binaries of 'normal' and 'abnormal'. This is challenging for psychoanalysis, which tends to consider the importance of identity development and fixity (Giffney & Watson, 2017), although Freud acknowledged we develop from a fluid experience of bisexuality and 'polymorphous perversity'. Dowling (2017) argues that queer becomes a new 'fetish', which scapegoats 'fixity'.

Polyamorists might critique the 'tyranny of the couple', but may polyamory become a new tyranny? I think back to a client, who feels unhappily caught in a spider's web of polyamorous relating; struggling to know who they should be to whom and when, but identifying as modern, open and tolerant, with polyamory fitting in to that identity. To their mind, monogamous relationships are 'ownership'.

But culture is in flux. The culture of individualism, capitalism, consumerism and immediacy may be changing. We see a rise in social movements and collective concern (as can be noted by the climate crisis movements). Marian O'Connor in 'Polyamory- a romantic solution to Wanderlust?' likewise refers to contemporary western culture as characterised by 'social reflexivity'. As the securities of the past (permanent jobs, affordable homes) have begun to erode, young people are engaged in constant choices about what to do, how to live and how to be. As O'Connor suggests, polyamory may offer a sense of community as a solution to increased loneliness and isolation. Besides, one might even go so far as to say that in some ways psychotherapists are polyamorous, albeit the feelings of love that the psychotherapist may have towards their patients are mostly fantasies ('Is Oedipus still Blind?')

Onel Brooks in 'Conversations outside the walls of the city: techniques, erotic love and the wings of desire in Phaedrus and psychotherapy' takes us back to the time when pederasty was a common form of relationship. In this special issue, we are concerned with diversity of relationships being accepted in time. What was previously taboo or pathologized may become accepted. However, this also reminds us that we should not forget that relationships previously accepted have become to be understood as unacceptable.

Temporality in psychotherapy

I would say that psychoanalysis has never been 'romantic'. It has always challenged notions of 'unconditional love', drawn attention to the presence of hate as well as love in relationships, and observed the existence of fantasy in relationships. We might even say that psychoanalysis is 'post-romantic'. However, I agree with many psychoanalytic theories in stating that relationships *are* important, particularly the quality of relationships. Attachment research and neuroscience have robustly shown this to be so (Music, 2016). Good relationships provide security. We may refer to secure and insecure attachments. Relationships have meaning, they have history, they have a function. They are complex, full of conflict, ebbs and flows. Do we permit ourselves the time to understand relationships, and our experience of love and hate; our common unhappiness? It is not for psychotherapists to judge whether the client's unhappiness is a common one or not, or what should be their common unhappiness. It is not the form of the relationships that matters as much as the quality of them. But, how might we as psychotherapists encourage exploration of the meaning of a relationship or relationships, without being accused of being old-fashioned, moralistic, wasting time in talking too much, or making radical suggestions?

A couple of the papers refer to Bion's advice to psychotherapists to work 'without memory or desire'. The psychotherapist should patiently wait 'until a pattern "evolves"' (Bion, 1970, p. 124). However, it is naïve to think that as psychotherapists we can exclude our own memory and desire from the consulting room. Psychoanalytic theory is saturated with assumptions, particularly around gender and sexuality, with clear binary assumptions around male and female, masculinity and femininity, heterosexuality and homosexuality, active and passive. These are being challenged within psychoanalysis (e.g. Hertzmann & Newbigin, 2019). Although psychoanalysis once was, and can still be, subversive and radical (Freud certainly was in his day), it can all too readily be applied in a conservative way. We know the importance of using supervision and our own personal therapy to work through our countertransference and be aware of our own blind spots. Paola Valerio's 'Is Oedipus still blind?' is an interesting addition to this collection of papers, as it considers the therapist's own possible erotic desire for the patient, which is seldom thought about.

If the client wants to understand their relationships and their meaning, it takes time. However, we live in a culture where many have limited patience for reflection. We may still do meaningful work when pressed for time ('Is Oedipus still Blind?'), but we may be faced with the hesitancy of clients to spend time on reflection, rather than find solutions. As Helen Gilbert in 'Should Love be Unconditional' described in the support group, there was some impatience on the part of members regarding finding a solution to estrangement of family relationships, rather than understanding them, interrupting those who were taking too much time talking.

Temporality is a feature of psychoanalytic psychotherapy, concerned as it is with the relation of the past to the present. Not only is this relevant in terms of transference, which may take some time to understand, but also to what French psychoanalysts refer to as *aprés-coup* (Birksted-Breen, 2016), where temporality moves from present to past, in that the present has an influence on the past. Much of the work of interpretation in psychotherapy may have reference to *aprés-coup*, in that working through issues of the present (here-and-now) has an influence on working through the past. Birksted-Breen (2016) argues that you cannot have one without the other, in that an interpretation, which may be a transference interpretation, has an influence on reorganising the client's understanding of the past. This is suggested in Sally Parsloe's and Onel Brooks' papers, where the example cases involved not only understanding the meaning of relationships in the here-and-now, but its significance for understanding and working through the client's past. In 'Conversations outside the walls of the city: techniques, erotic love and the wings of desire in Phaedrus and psychotherapy' the therapist begins with a reference to the client's father, when the client talks about her relationship to older men. Here time is also significant, with the client stating that there are 'so many men and such little time' (special issue page number). It was noteworthy that the therapist could do so much, in such a short space of time. The timing of interpretations and how they are made are also important considerations as shown in Paola Valerio's 'Is Oedipus still Blind?'.

Final reflections

The papers all made stimulating and enriching reading. The call for papers for the special issue suggested a number of questions to be asked. The papers did not necessarily answer them; rather, they prompted exploration of thought in relation to practice, opening up space for further reflection. Psychoanalytic psychotherapy is not so much about providing answers, but rather, asking questions that facilitate greater understanding. It provides an important and necessary opportunity for introspection and reflection in the presence of, and in relationship with, an empathic and understanding other (akin to Bion's notion of reverie). In an age of immediacy, of polarised debates, and increased loneliness and alienation, we need more time for this.

Disclosure statement

No potential conflict of interest was reported by the author.

References

Bion, W. R. (1962). *Learning from experience*. New York: Basic Books.
Bion, W. R. (1970). *Attention and interpretation: A scientific approach to insights in psychoanalysis and groups*. London: Tavistock.
Birksted-Breen, D. (2016). *The work of psychoanalysis: Sexuality, time and the psychoanalytic mind*. Abingdon: Routledge.
Bollas, C. (2013). *The Freudian moment*. London: Karnac Books.

Dowling, L. (2017). Perversion and the problem of fluidity and fixity. In N. Giffney & E. Watson (Eds.), *Clinical encounters in sexuality: Psychoanalytic practice and queer theory* (pp. 123–144). Punctum Books: Earth, Milky Way.

Giffney, N., & Watson, E. (Eds.). (2017). *Clinical encounters in sexuality: Psychoanalytic practice and queer theory*. Punctum Books: Earth, Milky Way.

Gil, N. (2014). Loneliness: A silent plague that is hurting young people most. *The Guardian, 20*. Available from: https://www.theguardian.com/lifeandstyle/2014/jul/20/loneliness-britains-silent-plague-hurts-young-people-most

Hertzmann, L., & Newbigin, J. (2019). *Sexuality and Gender Now: Looking beyond heteronormativity*. Abingdon: Routledge.

Klein, M. (1946). Notes on some schizoid mechanisms. *International Journal of Psychoanalysis, 27*, 99–110.

Layton, L. (2011). Something to do with a girl named Marla Singer: Capitalism, narcissism, and therapeutic discourse in David Fincher's Fight Club. *Free Associations, 12*(2), 111–133.

Lemma, A. (2017). *The digital age on the couch: Psychoanalytic practice and new media*. Abingdon: Routledge.

Lewes, K. (2009). *Psychoanalysis and male homosexuality (20th anniversary edition)*. Plymouth: Jason Aronson.

Music, G. (2016). *Nurturing natures: Attachment and children's emotional, socio-cultural and brain development*. London: Psychology Press.

Nettleton, S. (2017). *The metapsychology of Christopher Bollas: An introduction*. Abingdon: Routedge.

Winnicott, D. W. (1960). The theory of the parent-infant relationship. *International Journal of Psychoanalysis, 41*, 585–595.

Winnicott, D. W. (1965). *The maturational processes and the facilitating environment: Studies in the theory of emotional development*. London: The Hogarth Press and the Institute of Psychoanalysis.

Winnicott, D. W. (1969). The use of an object. *International Journal of Psychoanalysis, 50*, 711–716.

Winnicott, D. W. (1971). *Playing and reality*. London: Tavistock.

Love, sex and psychotherapy in a post-romantic age: A commentary

Christopher Clulow

ABSTRACT

Post-romanticism can be viewed as an historical construct that can be applied to singular experiences as well as broad understandings of change in couple and family relationships. This commentary focuses on the former approach, building on the six papers in this special issue. Four interconnected themes are explored: the relationship between falling in love and partner choice; the pull of narcissism and push of relating present in every developing love relationship; the experience of loss involved in surrendering illusion; and an exploration of what love in the consulting room might look like. The broad conclusion arrived at is that stable and satisfying relationships are post-romantic in the sense that they have in common the capacity to engage with and develop from the many minor deaths associated with enduring love. This provides a definition of the task therapists are often asked to assist with by those seeking help for troubled relationships.

Post-romanticism and the therapeutic endeavour

The romantic movement, a literary, artistic, musical and intellectual phenomenon that spanned the late 18th to mid 19th centuries, emphasised the importance of emotion as an authentic source of authority. It espoused individualistic values, focusing on ever-changing internal states of consciousness and resisted constraints imposed by external circumstance. The movement is commonly understood as having been a reaction against the rationalism, reductionism and privilege associated with the Age of Enlightenment, and what was seen as a debasement of human life caused by the Industrial Revolution.

Echoes of the romantic movement are to be found in contemporary European perspectives on family and community relationships: love as the basis for partner choice, self-realization coming before commitment to others, anger about displacement, and anxiety about the impact the economic order is having on individuals and families. So, we might ask, in what sense can the current landscape of couple and family relationships be regarded as post-romantic?

The authors of this fascinating collection of papers – perhaps unsurprisingly given their profession – eschew taking a macroscopic snapshot of current social values and mores and opt to address this question from a phenomenological, developmental perspective. In particular, they attempt, rather ambivalently, to capture aspects of the nature of love as expressed through people's behaviour in different relational circumstances. I say 'ambivalently', since they share the view that it is a fool's errand to try to capture, define and theorise about the caprice's of human passion. But, as practitioners facing patients whose lives have been upended by their affective experiences, they – and we – have no alternative. We are asked to help people understand why their love relationships have gone awry. As this is one of the thorniest of human problems, from which no-one is exempt, the ideas that inform our practice are likely to be highly subjective. Nevertheless, the therapeutic endeavour may be post-romantic in the sense that psychotherapists work to enable patients to bear the loss associated with disillusionment. But we might also say that the endeavour is romantic in privileging emotion and valuing the authenticity of individual experience. Ambiguity and conflict form part of the territory.

Falling in love and partner choice

An assumption implicit in all the papers is that every stable couple relationship is post-romantic: while the heady passions generated by falling in love can drive partner choice and provide the momentum that enables individuals to commit to each other, they are not usually sustainable over time, and so must be succeeded by something acceptably more mundane if the relationship is to survive and flourish.

The romantic experience of being *in* love is intoxicating, crazy-making, distorting and destabilising. It is, as Anthony McSherry describes, a 'Jellybean' phenomenon, exciting us to chase shapes and shadows that may be no more than reflections of ourselves. The hormonal disturbances that come with it provide an addictive buzz that drives us to become obsessed with the object of our desire, allowing him or her to dominate our thoughts and govern our behaviour (Fishbane, 2013; Marazziti & Canale, 2004). This elixir distorts our vision. Like Shakespeare's love-stricken Queen Titania, we see not the reality of a Bottom who is everything Titania is not – a mule-headed peasant – but the hologram of everything we desire. Threaten to remove this image and we are afflicted by intense anxiety; remove it and we are plunged into the depths of despair. We know that most of the regions of the brain activated by romantic love share common neurological pathways with substance addiction, a condition not usually associated with the capacity to read social situations accurately and the exercise of good judgement (Bartels & Zeki, 2000; Fisher, Xu, Aron, & Brown, 2016). We might say, like Freud, that falling in love is akin to suffering from a temporary psychosis, a psychosis that has much in common with obsessional compulsive disorders and borderline states of mind (Tallis, 2005). It generates an idealization of self and other, packaged in an exclusive bubble, and strives to avoid the pin-prick of an alternative reality that will burst the fondly cultivated illusion – perhaps replacing Jellybean's illusory shadow with the otherness of the lion Anthony McSherry (in 'A phenomenology of love, thanks to Lacan, Miller, and Jellybean') refers to, whose language we cannot understand. The lion is to be hated and feared because it shatters the idealisation of self and others, threatening a kind of death – the death of an illusion.

The pursuit of short-term, serial sexual and love relationships, which no longer attracts the social censure of bygone days, may be viewed, then, as symptomatic of an addiction to the dopamine highs they can offer, and as an inability to give up on the illusion that there is a perfect match to be found if only one persists in the hunt for long enough. This illusion references back to Aristophanes' tongue in cheek myth of gender and sexual preference, told at Plato's Symposium to explain why we choose the partners we do. The myth described humans as male, female and androgynous spheres, each having two heads and two sets of limbs. As humans grew in strength they challenged the gods, and so Zeus ordered them to be cut in half to reduce their power. Love was then driven by the desire to be whole once more, to be reunited with one's other half, whether same or other sex, and this became the basis of partner choice. The illusion that there might be that perfect complement to the self may be facilitated by dating agencies supplying no end of candidates for the role. Given that humans can only process a limited number of choices without suffering from cognitive overload, the 'plenty more fish in the sea' message may increase rather than reduce the complexity of partner choice.

There is an alternate view. The biological anthropologist Helen Fisher (2016) understands sexual freedom in serial relationships as a rational process of mate selection, reflecting current values that encourage self-realization. From this perspective, partnerships are rigorously tested, sometimes to the point of destruction, as part of the process of finding a suitable mate. Marriage (or stable cohabitation) then becomes the destination, not the point of departure for this journey of discovery. This is in stark contrast to a central premise in developmental psychology: that we come to discover ourselves and the otherness of others through our relationship with them. This perspective, which also underlies psychoanalytic couple psychotherapy (see, for example, Morgan, 2019), focuses on the containment relationships can provide to enable individuals to withstand and learn from the hate as well as love associated with intimacy, a hate that comes from having illusions challenged.

We are indeed more likely to be drawn to potential partners who are similar to rather than different from us. Similarities in race, culture, outlook, values, education, interests and so on, are evident in the majority of partnerships, and partners these days are more likely to be judged on the basis of compatibility and companionability than on the bread-winning and homemaker skills that once they were: symmetry and similarity now feature more in partner choice than demarcation and difference. However, while we might specify what we are looking for in a partner we often don't quite know what we want, and so dating agencies might come to rely more on an algorithm of our past behaviour than on expressed preferences when choosing matches ('customers who chose this have also liked … ').

The pull of narcissism and the push of relating

The emphasis psychoanalytically informed couple psychotherapists place on Kleinian concepts, such as projective identification, similarly assumes an historically-rooted algorithm bias towards the pursuit of the familiar when choosing a partner – that the unconscious internal worlds of partners share similar dynamic features that draw them together, allowing them to alternate between set roles in enacting couple dramas that come from similar family-of-origin scripts. Anthony McSherry in 'A phenomenology of love, thanks to Lacan, Miller, and Jellybean' quotes Miller and Lacan as basing partner choice on the person we believe might best answer the question 'Who am I?'. The search for someone who will either define us, or be defined by us, is driven not by the search for a relationship but for a kind of merger, a safe haven or harbour that offers protection from the anticipated storm of setting out on a voyage of discovery. Psychoanalytic theories about partner choice have been generated in a context where relationships have been troubled, and they are often troubled precisely because partners make narcissistic assumptions about each other. The therapist's task is then to expose the shared unconscious phantasy – the illusion – that binds partners together in this constrictive hold. Development in their relationship is gauged in terms of movement along a continuum, a process aptly described by the subtitle of a book focusing on just this issue 'emerging from narcissism towards marriage' (Fisher, 1999). The progress of couple therapy can be assessed in similar terms.

In short, therapists are likely to agree that the quality and stability of partnerships are made rather than chosen. Work, mortgages, children, relatives, health, and friends are just some of the external factors that shape the ties binding couples together. So is the passage of time: a five-year-old relationship is very different from one of fifty years standing. These variables invite partners to refine and extend their repertoire of roles in relation to each other and to others outside their partnership. They interact with internal factors resulting from each individual's earlier experiences of intimate relationships to generate meanings; as the saying goes, it's not what is happening to you that is important, but what you think is happening to you. The point is that individuals and relationships are not fixed entities but changing dynamic structures. In the WEIRD world (western, educated, industrialised, rich and democratic), environmental factors place fewer constraints on the scope for individual development than is the case for the remaining 88% of the world's population (Otto & Keller, 2014), and so it may be that the internal environment holds greater sway. Whilst our earliest family experiences provide us with templates for adult relationships, these templates are not immutable, and may be less pliable than in cultures where collective values take precedence over those of the individual (although collective values can also assert a rigid hold). In the latter case, insulation from the experiences of others may render relational templates rigid, protecting against an historically-rooted fear that change will result in a collapse of internal configurations upon which self-identity has come to depend. It is in just these circumstances that couples often seek help.

Loss and change

Successful relationships might then be viewed as those where partners have not only survived but built on the process of losing their illusions, about themselves and each other. Therapy, likewise, might be viewed as a process of enabling disillusionment. The key experience here is one of loss, and the key prognostic factor is the capacity to engage with rather than turn away from loss.

One of the illusions that is hardest to give up for those who have struggled with difficult relationships in childhood is that of the 'happy family'. This illusion of unconditional love between family members, that Helen Gilbert's 'Should Love be Unconditional' articulates so clearly, constructs normal family life as one in which parents and children always love each other and brothers and sisters always get along. The more the image is relied upon to bolster security, the harder it is to give up. Moreover, the price of challenging the image, of departing from the family script, may be to become the family problem, resulting in a choice of accepting that role or being banished from the family group and the security it provides. The conditions for external security then come up against those governing an internal sense of security, which emanate from the authenticity and integrity of personal experience. This conflict is evident in the literature of the Romantic era, witness the novels of Jane Austen, and is one that we may be seeing today in relation to expressing sexual preference and gendered identity. In terms of dilemmas arising from the sense that love within families should be unconditional, the problem may lie with the illusion that family relationships are fixtures, children never grow up into adults, parents will always be needed by their offspring, and siblings have more in common than not. As 'Should Love be Unconditional' illustrates from those using the services of *Stand Alone*, and from those seeking individual help with family estrangement, the default emotion for those who are left may be anger, and for those who leave guilt. What unites them, and may jointly be defended against, is the experience of loss. Letting the past go when nothing can be changed, or when relationships once depended upon have become redundant, involves mourning the 'happy family' illusion and accepting a different reality.

Idealization is one means of maintaining illusions and avoiding engaging with loss. It involves the unconscious process of splitting and maintaining in separated compartments positive and negative object relations (internalised representations of relational experiences), along with the affects associated with them. As Sally Parsloe's 'Romance and Murder' asserts, chief amongst these are feelings of love and hate towards the same object (internal) or person (external). It is noteworthy that without exception the emotion of hate appears in this collection of papers on love.

Splitting is not necessarily a pathological process, and can provide a means of exploring and playing with relationship scenarios that generate high levels of anxiety. The fairy tales depicting forces of good and evil locked in conflict with each other, the games children play together to engage with potentially threatening situations, and the dramatic arts reflecting the preoccupations of adulthood, allow us to engage at one remove with these scenarios, reading our own experiences into their unfolding stories, allowing us to think about ourselves through thinking about them. Romantic and murderous feelings, as 'Romance and Murder' illustrates, go hand in hand, because the reality of the other – the person we allow ourselves to see once the scales of illusion fall from our eyes – challenges not only how we perceive them but also how we perceive ourselves. Facing these realities involves the loss of illusion. That is a kind of death, and, as the poet reminds us in relation to our own mortality, 'human kind cannot bear very much reality' (Eliot, 1935/1969, p. 172).

Can polyamory justifiably be understood in terms of defending against loss? Does it reflect a failure of surviving the loss involved in navigating oedipal conflicts, where the genitalization of infantile sexuality places attachment to mother in conflict with sexual rivalry with father, resulting in Freud's prediction (for men) that 'where they love they do not desire, and where they desire they do not love' (1912, p. 183)? Where, as Paola Valerio in 'Is Oedipus still blind?' asks, is Electra to provide a gender balance to the psychoanalytic narrative of sexual development? Is polyamory symptomatic of splitting sex and attachment needs, those hard-wired systems that some believe are essentially incompatible (Eagle, 2007)? Or have images of and allegiances to outdated family structures blinded us to the possibilities of a more generous vision of human intimacy and sexuality, one that does not expect a single individual to excel in a multiplicity of roles?

Marian O'Connor's 'Polyamory- a romantic solution to Wanderlust?' addresses the challenges facing psychoanalytic psychotherapists when much of their practice is informed by theories that assume monogamy as the norm. Breaking ranks with that assumption risks isolation, in much the same way as those in polyamorous relationships find themselves unsupported by kith and kin. Therapists meet those in polyamorous relationships when something is not working – there is a problem. On the one hand the problem may be defined as resistance to an emerging normality, one that no longer requires transgressing the monogamous contract through an act of infidelity for self-fulfilment, and accepts that one person cannot meet all the needs their partner may have. On the other, these arrangements may unconsciously be intended to defend against the fear that past loss and trauma will be resurrected if all one's emotional eggs are placed in the same basket, an arrangement that in such circumstances can have the unintended consequence of precipitating precisely what is trying to be avoided. As Marian O'Connor notes, there are challenges to psychotherapists here: we may unintentionally dilute the value of the service we provide by forming a quasi-polyamorous system with our patients when we become part of the network of therapists supporting them. Even when operating alone, and perhaps especially in these circumstances, we may offer a kind of intimacy to individuals that rivals and replaces what properly belongs in their marriage or partnership. In such circumstances we face the risk of simply re-enacting and reinforcing the problem for which our patients are seeking help. As with other questions raised in the course of a therapy, we may need to develop a polyamorous state of mind in the sense of remaining open to learning from our patients and helping them find solutions that work for them.

Love in the consulting room

What is our stance as psychoanalytically informed psychotherapists to the ubiquity of love, a word that surfaces in multiple contexts as noun, adjective and verb? Onel Brooks, in 'Conversations outside the walls of the city: techniques, erotic love and the wings of desire in Phaedrus and psychotherapy', cautions, none of us is immune to its force field, however determinedly, like Phaedrus and Socrates, we forge defensive alliances to explain rather than to experience its power, or to pursue the narcissistic goal of appropriating what we most admire in others. Like the apocryphal group of therapists passing from this world into the next and being faced with a signpost to the Garden of Eden or to the Lecture on the Garden of Eden we may nervously opt for the latter.

Therapy relationships combine intimacy and formality in a rare and sometimes uneasy marriage. In classical terms we encounter the participant-observer dilemma when we try to distinguish between our countertransference to patients, an essential tool we rely upon for decoding their unconscious communications, and our transference to patients, which is essentially about us and not them. Paola Valerio in 'Is Oedipus still blind?' explores this territory in arresting detail, challenging the gender bias implicit in some of our favoured theories and inviting honesty in acknowledging our own feelings, especially those of erotic desire. In contemporary terms we are in the territory of intersubjectivity, where we and our patients each contributes to creating an experience, consciously and unconsciously, from which both might learn. Therapy is more about exploring than explaining, and both parties have to be open to themselves and each other for the venture to succeed.

That does not mean we are without boundaries. If we move from the passive experience of 'being in love' to the active process of loving another person, warts and all, what might love in the consulting room look like? Attachment theorists tend to describe romantic love in terms of three interacting behavioural systems: attachment, caregiving and sexuality. When it comes to thinking about the therapist-patient couple it is the attachment-caregiving system that features prominently, with the therapist often being construed as an attachment figure for the patient, providing the secure base from which it becomes safe for the patient to venture out and explore the world of relationships. Therapists have drawn on this paradigm to inform psychoanalytic work with adult couple relationships, sharing empirical frameworks derived from developmental psychology as well as psychoanalysis (Clulow, 2001, 2014). Inevitably, this approach looks backwards in time, regarding early family experiences as the forge from which relationships in later life are shaped. Oddly, the sexual behavioural system is the one least explored, and this may be relevant to Paola Valerio's observation that viewers of *In Treatment* tend to be more comfortable discussing the case of Mia than Laura. Even among couple therapists there can be reticence about entering this unpredictable and potentially chaotic realm, perhaps because of the anxiety it can cause (Kahr, 2009). It may feel safer for us to assume, and so to interpret, that sex is being used in the service of attachment than to engage with erotic feelings that have been generated intersubjectively.

Which leads me to a fourth realm constituting adult love relationships: intersubjectivity. Stern (2004) saw this as a distinct behavioural system with similar activating and deactivating properties as the other three. For him this system was driven by the need to share with others, and to define or maintain the cohesion of the self. It resembles the sociable, affiliative system described by Bowlby (1969), which drives children to form relationships with others not simply for comfort and reassurance but also for play. Intersubjectivity permeates attachment, caregiving and sexuality, and it is questionable whether it can be regarded as a distinct behavioural system in terms comparable to the other three. Nevertheless, it is of great relevance for psychotherapists, whose role includes creating the conditions that facilitate play, as well as sharing affiliative enjoyment with patients and engaging with unconscious intersubjective processes.

In our post-romantic attempts to understand the multifaceted dimensions of love we often fall back on definition – the naming of parts – as I have done in depicting a Venn image of four separate but interacting, and occasionally converged, behavioural systems. The authors in this issue have drawn on philosophers and psychoanalysts to describe aspects of love and the dynamics of desire, edging us towards an appreciation and understanding of this most complex of human emotions. The 'labyrinth of misunderstanding' that Anthony McSherry cites in exploring the phenomenology of love is precisely what brings individuals, couples and families to therapy. So it behoves us as psychotherapists to be as clear as we can about the experiences we encounter, and their relationship to what we might consider to be a love relationship.

All the contributors share the view that romanticism can be the enemy of love insofar as it insulates against relating, preventing the testing of our perceptions, beliefs and assumptions against those of others. Insulation is often the product of love relationships having gone wrong earlier in life, illusion providing a protective buffer against the fear of re-encountering past hurt or trauma. Psychotherapy aims to offer a safe environment for taking the risk of testing these realities, but it can only do so if we as psychotherapists appreciate that the process is two-way. We also take a risk when testing our realities against those who consult us, and while we are better protected because of the asymmetry of the therapy relationship, the onus on us to be available and open to influence is all the greater because of that asymmetry.

I have been drawn to the idea that love is akin to the spark of positive energy, capable of being triggered by just a smile, that synaptically connects neurones and releases neuropeptides that not only make you feel good but nourish networks of interconnectivity in the brain. Repeated connections reinforce these pathways; neglect results in their atrophy. Transferring this image to human relationships, love has been defined as a 'micro moment of positivity resonance' (Fredrickson, 2016, p. 852) where shared positive emotion and a sense of mutual care forge an experience of connection. For me this sits well with Winnicott's (1967) perception of the therapeutic task as 'mirroring' explicit and implicit communications, not in the sense of echoing such transmission but making visible what was previously unseen, validating the experience, and making it available for review. What was previously unseen includes negative as well as positive feelings; love in this context is not a 'love-in', but contains hate. This is not a one-off process but a repeated sequence, comprising a multitude of repeated love experiences.

Drawing on developmental psychology and neuroscience for an explication of love may be like standing too far outside the walls of Onel Brooks city to remain connected with the passions of the heart. We can never be sure when working with prose and passion that we have the balance right. But we short-change ourselves and our patients if we lose sight of either heart or mind, and the significance of the objects to which they become attached. The act of loving is never conflict-free.

Disclosure statement

No potential conflict of interest was reported by the author.

References

Bartels, A., & Zeki, S. (2000). The neural basis of romantic love. *NeuroReport, 11* (17), 3829–3834.

Bowlby, J. (1969). *Attachment.* London: Hogarth and Institute of Psychoanalysis.

Clulow, C. (ed.). (2001). *Adult attachment and couple psychotherapy. The 'secure base' in practice and research.* London: Brunner-Routledge.

Clulow, C. (2014). Attachment, affect regulation and couple psychotherapy. In D. Scharff & J. Savege Scharff (Eds.), *Psychoanalytic couple therapy. Foundations of theory and practice* (pp. 44–58). London: Karnac.

Eagle, M. (2007). Attachment and sexuality. In D. Diamond, S. Blatt, & J. Lichtenberg (Eds.), *Attachment and sexuality* (pp. 27–50). New York: Analytic Press.

Eliot, T. S. (1935/1969). *Burnt Norton, four quartets. The Complete Poems and Plays of T.S. Eliot.* London: Faber and Faber.

Fishbane, M. (2013). *Loving with the brain in mind. Neurobiology and couple therapy.* New York: Norton.

Fisher, H. (2016). *Anatomy of love. A natural history of mating, marriage, and why we stray.* New York: Norton.

Fisher, H. E., Xu, X., Aron, A., & Brown, L. L. (2016). Intense, passionate, romantic love: A natural addiction? How the fields that investigate romance and substance abuse can inform each other. *Front Psychol, 7,* 687. Published 2016 May 10

Fisher, J. (1999). *The uninvited guest. Emerging from narcissism towards marriage.* London: Karnac.

Frederickson, B. (2016). Love. Positivity resonance as a fresh, evidence-based perspective on an age-old topic. In L. Feldman Barrett, M. Lewis, & J. Haviland-Jones (Eds.), *Handbook of emotions* (pp. 847–858). New York: Guilford Press.

Freud, S. (1912). *On the universal tendency to debasement in the sphere of love. S.E, 11* (pp. 177–190). London: Hogarth.

Kahr, B. (2009). Psychoanalysis and sexpertise. In C. Clulow (Ed.), *Sex, attachment and couple psychotherapy. Psychoanalytic perspectives* (pp. 1–24). London: Karnac.

Marazziti, D., & Canale, D. (2004). Hormonal changes when falling in love. *Psychoneuroendocrinology, 29,* 931–936.

Morgan, M. (2019). *A couple state of mind. Psychoanalysis of couples and the tavistock relationships model.* Abingdon: Routledge.

Otto, H., & Keller, H. (2014). eds. *Different faces of attachment. Cultural variations on a human need.* Cambridge: Cambridge University Press.

Stern, D. (2004). *The present moment in psychotherapy and everyday life.* New York: Norton.

Tallis, F. (2005). *Love sick.* London: Arrow.

Winnicott, D. (1967). Mirror role of mother and family in child development. In D. Winnicott (Ed.), *Playing and reality* (pp. 111–118). London: Tavistock.

Index